Insights into H

Francis Hervey Bodman
MD, DPM, FFHom

Edited for publication by

Anita Davies
MB, BS, MRCP, DCH, DObstRCOG, FFHom

and

Robin Pinsent
OBE, MA, MD, FRCGP, FRACGP, MFHom

BEACONSFIELD PUBLISHERS LTD
Beaconsfield, Bucks, England

© Janet Bodman 1990

British Library Cataloguing in Publication Data
Bodman, Francis Hervey, *1900–1980*
  Insights into homoeopathy –
  (The Beaconsfield Homoeopathic Library; no. 12)
  1. Medicine. Homeopathy
  I. Title. II. Davies, Anita III. Pinsent, Robin, *d. 1987*
  615.5'32

ISBN 0–906584–28–0

Phototypeset by Gem Graphics, Trenance, Mawgan Porth, Cornwall in 10 on 12 point Times.
Printed in Great Britain at The Bath Press, Avon.

Foreword

Frank Bodman's professional publications divided more or less equally between general and psychological medicine and homoeopathy. A number of his papers were translated into foreign languages, including one wartime paper that was 'pirated' by the German propaganda radio. As a competent linguist he also translated the works of others, notably Dr J. Baur of Lyons, whose *Petite Histoire de l'Organon et de ses Metamorphoses* appeared in 1975. He was in demand as a lecturer on subjects as far apart as botany and social science, and was invited to write the obituary of many of the distinguished homoeopathic physicians of his day. An interesting biographical sketch of him appeared in the January 1990 issue of the *British Homoeopathic Journal*.

Frank's approach to the problems of child care and delinquency was liberal, and in respect of homoeopathy he had no illusions. While he looked hopefully towards the ultimate acceptance of homoeopathy as part of medicine as a whole, he was not blind to its own imperfections.

In his Presidential Address to the Faculty of Homoeopathy in 1975 he said, '. . . The minority group is separated from the traditional community by the differences in its beliefs and convictions. The group is bound together by its beliefs, which become organised into a dogmatic system which is fiercely defended against the disbelief of the world. The consequence of this self-imposed isolation is that any contacts with the outside world are aggressive. Not only do these aggressive contacts provoke a corresponding response from the unbelieving world, but there is a well-known tendency for the aggression to strike not only outwards but inwards within the group. The phenomenon of the aggression directed both inwards and outwards of the minority group was well exemplified in the earliest days of homoeopathy, and has been a feature of its history and development in nearly every country in the world.'

Those who have had an opportunity to read much of Frank Bodman's work, in manuscript, in typescript and finally in reprint form, cannot fail to be impressed by the breadth and balance of his thinking and the pains he took in the preparation of material to be published. Editing and rearrangement of manuscripts, meticulous correction of typescripts and top copies were the rule, and comprehensive reference lists bore witness to that greatly extended memory capability that is the hallmark of the successful homoeopath.

We can see him as an able and competent practitioner of conventional medicine with a scientific turn of mind, although he always maintained that medical practice is an art as well as a science. He would appear distinguished in any company. He was, however, possessed of something more – the breadth of mind which enabled him to look at homoeopathy as a subject to which proper scientific scrutiny could and should legitimately be applied. Had he written his own book, this is surely the case he would have made.

New concepts in medicine, unless they derive from research within a specialty, are not readily accepted. The pressures that led to psychiatry occurred during World War I. New dimensions were added to orthopaedics and manipulative surgery by the use – and the competition of – the osteopath and chiropractor. Ideas developing in the lay field are looked at particularly askance until the pressures build up to overwhelm professional conservatism. As we enter the 21st century, acupuncture and hypnosis are very close to the point at which the barrier of professional orthodoxy will be broken.

So it is with homoeopathy. To the conventionally-trained beholder there is as yet no unassailable proof of the microdose effect in terms of reversal of pathology, by which he is accustomed to measure the success or failure of a therapeutic agent. Such effects as are observed are conveniently ascribed to 'suggestion', though the mechanism of this, too, remains unexplained.

In recent years the pressures towards what is now called holistic medicine, complementary to the teaching in medical schools, have built up steadily. Those concerned have for the most part been non-medical scientists, research workers in allied fields, and – damning in the eyes of the orthodox – informed lay people who share an almost intuitive feeling that reductionist medicine does not provide all the answers to problems experienced by whole organisms. Knowing how genes control enzymes may tell us little about the ways in which enzymes mediate the patterns of living and bodily functions.

Unlike some of his contemporaries, Frank Bodman was eminent in fields outside homoeopathy, practising orthodox psychiatry and conducting research into mental disorder and disability. In the chapters which follow we have tried to distil his philosophy and practice from the large body of published and unpublished material that he left.

One of our aims in editing this work has been to introduce homoeopathy as it is practised today to orthodox medical practitioners whose minds remain open to new ideas – though the idea of *similia similibus curentur* (the imperative form: 'Let likes be cured by likes') is as old as Paracelsus. We have kept to Bodman's original texts as far as possible. In those places where overlap remains, it derives from his remarkable and enriching ability to look at the same subject from many different angles.

We have not followed him in his meticulous and almost obsessional preoccupation with references. His original work is embedded in a matrix composed of the thoughts and writings of doctors and scientists in many disciplines – few can have read so widely and selected so critically. Those embarking on a career in homoeopathic medicine may wish to study his writings in fuller detail. We hope that this book might act as a stimulus to those who may be encouraged to do so.

A.E.D.
R.J.F.H.P.

Dr Pinsent died suddenly on Christmas Day 1987, having just agreed the final form this book should take. He was a remarkable person, and shared Frank's meticulous interest in detail.

A.E.D.

Contents

Chapter 1

Wider Issues

I was under no pressure from my family to become a homoeopathic doctor. My father, who was a gold medallist and trained in medicine at St Bartholomew's Hospital, London, was very careful to leave me freedom of choice in this matter, so that after qualification I spent two years in a variety of residential posts in a teaching hospital before coming to London to learn homoeopathy. After a year's study I returned to my home town of Bristol and was engaged in general practice for ten years before qualifying as a consultant.

I found the postgraduate study of homoeopathy very stimulating. I had sufficient experience of orthodox medicine to appreciate what could and could not be done, and my introduction to homoeopathic medicine as a resident at The Royal London Homoeopathic Hospital opened up new avenues and provided new tools; a whole range of illnesses became treatable, where before I had accepted from my teachers a therapeutic nihilism. This of course was a long time ago, before barbiturates, sulphonamides, antibiotics or steroids were discovered.

One of the most fascinating aspects of homoeopathy is the focus on the individual patient. The target is the patient himself and the mobilisation of his defence mechanisms, rather than a frontal attack on the infecting agent or diseased organ. I do not have to worry whether the infecting agent is resistant to this or that antibiotic, or whether it is a virus unaffected by any known antibiotic. I do not have to subject my patient to the collection of tissue specimens, painful and even dangerous as these can be, because I am not so concerned with his liver, or kidney, or testes, but rather with his total reaction; and his total reaction includes not only his response to physical stimuli – heat, cold, damp, movement, and rest – but also his mental reaction to social stimuli, his irritability or his apathy, his excitement or despair, his retreat into silence or his excursion into loquacity. These 'mental' symptoms are regarded by the homoeopath as valuable indicators in choosing the remedy. Not only are the primary behaviour reactions to social stimuli important, such as desire for solitude or craving for company, need for consolation or aversion from sympathy; of great importance, too, are the physical consequences of emotion, the colic after an argument, the frequency after an altercation, the menorrhagia after a fright, the diarrhoea before an interview, the amenorrhoea after a change of job.

This is the field of psychosomatic medicine. The homoeopath can observe in the earliest stages – and treat – the reactions and responses which, fixed and frozen into habitual responses, become the basis of psychosomatic illnesses such as asthma, eczema, gastric ulcer, ulcerative colitis and various disorders of the menstrual cycle. Further, since his objective is to treat the patient as a whole, he can hope for a cure, rather than the suppression of a troublesome symptom.

What do the antihistamines do but counteract the end result of the allergic processes (the release of histamine), and with what side effects will the patient have to pay for this measure of relief? The homoeopath, in selecting the appropriate constitutional remedy, expects to desensitise the allergic patient to all allergens – not just the specific allergen, as for example the pollen in hay fever. Again, the various alkalis and buffer substances aim to neutralise the overproduction of acid by the patient liable to peptic ulcers. The fundamental dysfunction is the overproduction of hydrochloric acid, which is a constitutional dysfunction, as may be deduced from its association with the different blood groups and the hereditary factors. To tackle the patient with a liability to peptic ulceration, a constitutional treatment is required.

Aspirin may be as effective as cortisone in relieving the pain of rheumatic disease, but it cannot be claimed that it is a cure. Here again constitutional factors play a part, whether the patient suffers from gout, acute rheumatism, arthritis or fibrositis; but in each case we have to bear in mind the individual patient and his response to the particular stimuli which trigger off the symptoms of his illness, whether they are climatic or mechanical or emotional. Antihistamines, alkalis or aspirin are so much first aid, and surely our objectives should be more profound.

Dr Yudkin, in a paper in *The Lancet* entitled 'Six Children with Coughs', spoke of the need of a second diagnosis: 'Why did the patient consult the doctor?', and demonstrated the importance of what might be called 'second aid'. For the homoeopath, a third and further diagnosis is essential – a diagnosis in terms of remedy sensitivity: 'To which remedy will this patient be most sensitive?' This will be discovered by matching the totality of his symptoms with the symptoms produced in healthy persons by the corresponding remedy. This pharmacological diagnosis is essential for treatment and constitutes the 'third aid'.

This pharmacological expertise involves learning. The additional pharmacology is more precise, more detailed and more intimate than the materia medica that the medical student learns, or the knowledge he acquires in practice from the daily flood of literature sent by pharmaceutical firms. While the homoeopathic materia medica is an extensive one, its total is not so great as the modern pharmacopoeia, with its hundreds of antibiotics, analgesics, sedatives, tranquillisers, purgatives, hypotensives, anticoagulants, steroids, diuretics and bronchodilators, many of them with synthetic names as well as official alibis.

Personally, I found the best plan in learning the homoeopathic materia medica was to concentrate on mastering the symptomatology of a dozen well-known and frequently prescribed remedies, and after that to add to my repertoire bit by bit.

Recently, I carried out a survey in my outpatient department to find out how many homoeopathic remedies I had used in three months. I found I had made use of a hundred remedies in that time, but that only twenty of them had been used on more than five occasions.

In learning new methods and new techniques, the keeping of accurate records is important. This is true whatever one's interests may be, whether photography, birdwatching or collecting fossils; for we learn by our mistakes and failures, and by checking back we can see where we failed to give the right exposure, or to note the colour of the bird's leg or the marking on the fossil shell.

Note-taking in homoeopathic medicine is essential, and it is important not to cramp oneself. I do not think it is possible to list the essentials on the National Health Service record card, and I think it advisable to use a quarto folder, at least, for each patient. While it will be important to list all the symptoms elicited from the patient in practice, prescriptions will probably be based on some half-dozen significant symptoms. I suggest that these should be underlined. If you have made a successful prescription you will have reinforced your memory on the salient features of that particular remedy. If on the other hand you have missed the bull's eye (and 'outers' are rarely of any use in homoeopathy), then a revision of your list will be illuminating.

Increasing familiarity with the remedies will enable you to reach the point when you recognise the remedy picture as the patient walks into your surgery – so that you will recognise Mr Lycopodium, Mrs Sepia, Miss Pulsatilla and Master Chamomilla at a glance, and only a few questions will be necessary to confirm your identification. Just as the field botanist recognises the buttercup or the daisy at a glance and does not need to resort to an identification key, so the experienced homoeopath recognises the remedy types without having to look up his reference books. We can all tell old Mrs Smith from her back view fifty yards down the street, but we might be hard put to give the police an accurate description of her individual features. We recognise her as a whole.

As you acquire a deeper knowledge of your materia medica, you will find fresh interest in reading the orthodox medical journals. For example, the *British Medical Journal* and *The Lancet* have published articles on 'Monday head', which you will recognise as the symptoms described in the provings of the nitrate we call Glonoine; or you may have noted a communication on an epileptic patient, who was found to have taken pennyroyal as an abortifacient; or the dramatic case of renal failure following fungus poisoning, with its relation to the homoeopathic provings of Agaricus.

Moreover, as you acquire more confidence in your skill as a homoeopathic prescriber, you will be relieved of the anxieties attendant on the prescription of the powerful modern drugs, and free yourself from the responsibilities of occasioning the iatrogenic illnesses that they may induce.

In this respect the current journals present an alarming picture from time to time: papers on drug-induced gastrointestinal bleeding caused by anticoagulants given prophylactically after a coronary thrombosis; hepatitis caused by the amine oxidase inhibitors prescribed for depression, to quote only two examples. Of course these are accidents that happen to a small minority of patients, but they unfortunately illustrate the range of individual variation of response to drugs – the cardinal tenet of homoeopathic prescribing.

Apart from the negative advantages of the absence of serious side effects, you will enjoy the positive advantages of being equipped to tackle problems of patients that up to now were beyond the range of relief. I call to mind two examples, one a schoolboy working for his examinations who was prostrated one day a week with severe migraine, a year ago. He has passed in six subjects and has not had a headache for several months. Or again, a naval officer with very severe lichen planus staining his skin and limbs the characteristic violet colour over large areas, and causing intolerable itching. Six months treatment, without any external application, has resulted in almost complete relief.

I quote these cases not to boast of any special skill, but to illustrate the possibilities inherent in homoeopathic practice. Both patients were relieved with well-known and frequently prescribed homoeopathic remedies. Furthermore, the prescription of the homoeopathic remedy does not depend on the pathological or bacteriological report.

A disturbing feature of modern medicine is the appearance of new diseases. The report from Scotland of acute paralytic illnesses which were not due to polio is an illustration. A hundred and sixty-eight cases were reported which, though resembling polio, were caused by Cox-sackie viruses, mumps, leptosporosis or loupingill. The emergence of new 'virus' diseases is a possible result of the disturbance of balance caused by improved living conditions and immunisations. Whatever the cause of the virus, the homoeopath will be guided in his prescription by the patient's symptoms, not necessarily by the offending virus.

The basic principles underlying homoeopathic medicine equip the practitioner to deal with new illnesses. Hahnemann showed the way when he recommended the group of remedies likely to be indicated in the cholera epidemics that invaded Europe in the 1830s and 1840s, with a very significant reduction in mortality.

Chapter 2

Samuel Hahnemann

To appreciate the origins of homoeopathy we must get out of our cars; we must turn out our black bags and remove the blood pressure apparatus, antibiotics, etc. Going back only a century will take us no further than Florence Nightingale and the beginning of the professionally-trained nurse. We must also forget all bacteriology, anaesthetics, radiology, a good deal of our pathology, the germ theories of Pasteur and the cellular pathology of Virchow.

Two hundred years ago, when confronted with a patient, our first objective was not to transfuse him but to bleed him – even laymen carried lancets for this purpose. Louis Phillipe, the French king, always carried a spring lancet with him and used it on his staff if they became ill. Indeed, it was considered criminal negligence not to bleed a patient. Goethe, when over eighty, after a serious haemorrhage, was treated with a prolonged venesection. We would have been taught that most diseases were due to an excess of blood or plethora, or else to disease substances circulating in the blood. These acridities had to be cleaned out by venesections, cuppings, by giving emetic and purgative medicines, and by making the patient sweat and salivate profusely. A robust constitution was necessary to survive an illness and its treatment two centuries ago.

Samuel Hahnemann (1775–1843) came from a family of painters on porcelain at the famous Meissen factory, set up near Dresden by the Elector of Saxony, Augustus the Strong. Augustus was a fanatical collector of Chinese porcelain, and once exchanged a regiment of dragoons for a set of forty-eight vases. In the end, when the Treasury of Saxony was running dry, Augustus employed a young refugee alchemist to make gold. When the young alchemist failed he was set the task of making porcelain, and in this he was eventually successful. The factory at Meissen was established and artists were invited to work there. Among these was the father of Dr Hahnemann.

The Seven Years War began a year after Samuel was born. Frederick of Prussia occupied Dresden that autumn and looted the factory; many of the artists were forcibly transferred to Berlin, where the Prussian King was setting up his own rival factory. It was not until Samuel was eight years old that the Prussians relaxed their grip on the Meissen factory, and in the next few years there were many changes of management. The factory artists were sent on a tour of European factories to search for inspiration, and a French artist was introduced to meet the competition from Sèvres.

In those first eight years Samuel probably experienced poverty and hunger. We know that his father was unable to afford school fees, and it is clear that these experiences left an indelible impression on him. In later years, when advising his pupils about fees, he reminded them that they had to look after themselves and their families. He recommended cash fees and no credit.

When Samuel was fifteen his father made his 'submissive and most obedient' petition to his Serene Highness, Gracious Prince and Master, that his son should be admitted to the Prince's school at Meissen. There he came under the influence of a remarkable tutor, Magister Müller, and in that school he remained, half pupil, half usher, until he was twenty.

By breaking away from traditional Lutheranism, Hahnemann's father freed his son from orthodoxy, pedagogy and disciplinarian control. For the young German intellectual the constraints of feudalism were an incitement to withdraw into himself – to find compensation in professional activity, in science and in culture. Hahnemann gives us no clue to the motives behind his choice of medicine as a profession. All we know is that on leaving school his farewell dissertation was on the wonderful construction of the human hand.

We know he had a heroic conception of the physician and the nurse – 'two people chosen by God, thrown into the battle at its hardest, like forlorn sentries close to the attacking enemy with no relief. They strive to attain a citizen's crown amidst fatally poisonous atmospheres, overcome by anguished cries and dying moans.' This does not resemble the classical picture of the Garden of Aesculapius – cool, calm and leisurely – but rather forecasts the picture of the bearded doctor in the country cottage.

But if this was Hahnemann's conception of a doctor's life before he began his studies, he must have had a rather different initiation when he began his life's work at Leipzig University. He had been given free passes to the lectures on medicine by a Dresden doctor, but the university professors had neither clinic nor hospital at their disposal. Their lectures dealt with the theories and systems of medicine, but there was no opportunity for practical experience.

He moved on to Vienna, where he worked in a hospital under Dr Quarin, physician-in-ordinary to the Empress Maria Theresa, where he had opportunities not only in hospital practice but in a fashionable private practice. Quarin recommended him as a family physician to the newly-appointed Governor of Transylvania, and during the time of this Hungarian appointment Hahnemann saw many cases of malaria.

He wrote his MD thesis on cramp. This was accepted at the University of Erlangen when he was twenty-four. The next five years were spent in a search for an appointment that would support him and his family, and at the same time afford him sufficient leisure to acquire further knowledge.

He was dissatisfied with the results of the practice of medicine as it was currently taught. At the age of twenty-nine he published a little work, 'Directions for the Complete Cure of Old Wounds and Indolent Ulcers' (note the word 'complete'). He writes, 'The majority of physicians refuse to treat this condition and leave it to the barber surgeon – to shepherds and to hangmen – surely more from ignorance than disgust.' But he adds, 'He who has had as many opportunities as I to make obser-vations . . . who is induced by his desire for the welfare of his fellow beings to think and act for himself, he who like myself feels hatred for . . . any kind of recognition or great name and who eagerly endeavours to act and think independently . . . will see excellent results, which is the greatest reward an honest physician can expect.' Here is the freethinker coming to the fore. He goes on to write, 'Almost all our knowledge of the healing properties of natural products, as well as artificial products, is derived from the crude applications of the ordinary man.'

Further disillusionment was in store. In 1792 the Emperor Leopold II of Austria died suddenly – this monarch had raised high hopes of preventing a threatened war and his death was a national tragedy. Hahnemann was convinced from the medical bulletins that the specialists had killed him by four venesections in twenty-four hours, and did not hesitate to communicate his opinions to the press.

Were the obstacles to the attainment of simplicity and certainty in practical medicine insurmountable? 'After the discovery of the weakness and misconceptions of my teachers and books I sank into a state of morbid indignation . . . I was about to believe that the whole science was of no avail and incapable of improvement.'

'My sense of duty would not easily allow me to treat the unknown state of my suffering brethren with these unknown medicines. The thought of becoming in this way a murderer . . . was most terrible to me, so terrible and disturbing that I wholly gave up my practice in the first years of my married life. I scarcely treated anybody for fear of injuring him.'

'But then children were born to me, several children, and after a time serious illnesses occurred which in tormenting and endangering my children made it even more painful . . . that I could not with any sense of assurance procure help for them. I gave myself up to my own individual cogitations and determined to fix no goal for my considerations until I should have arrived at a decisive conclusion.'

Perhaps the young doctor was in the throes of a depressive attack, but he was not alone. Listen to that most famous psychiatrist, Freud: 'I have even given up my lectures this year in order not to talk about things I do not yet understand. I have become a therapist against my will.' Freud describes himself as isolated, stagnant, resigned. He wrote, 'Ideas whirl through my head, which promise to explain everything and to connect the normal and the pathological, and then they disappear again – and then one strenuous night last week, the barriers suddenly lifted, the veils dropped and it was possible to see all the way. Everything fell into place – the cogs meshed – the thing really seemed to be a machine which in a moment would run itself.'

A similar process had taken place in Hahnemann's mind a century before. In 1790, translating Cullen's *Materia Medica*, he criticised the famous Scottish physician's opinion on the mode of action of Peruvian bark – the source of quinine. Hahnemann had already been interested in malarial infections when he was practising in Hungary. He was familiar with Sydenham's researches with the Peruvian bark brought back to Europe by the Jesuit Fathers; and how Sydenham had differentiated the malarial from the non-malarial fevers by their response to treatment with quinine. He had already observed that substances which produced some kind of fever (such as very strong coffee, pepper, arnica, ignatia bean or arsenic) had some effect on these malarial infections. As an experiment he took a large dose of Peruvian bark twice daily; in brief, all the symptoms usually associated with malaria, yet without the actual rigor, appeared in succession. Hahnemann's interpretation was that the Peruvian bark, used as a remedy for malaria, acts because it can produce symptoms similar to malaria in healthy people.

In the next year, translating another materia medica, he made the generalisation that all substances stimulating a counter-irritation and artificial fever, if administered shortly before the attack, are deterrent to malaria and similar fevers.

It was another five years before he published his essay on a 'New Principle for Ascertaining the Curative Powers of Drugs'. In this paper he pleads for the investigation of the effects of remedies by experiments on the healthy human body. 'Every effective remedy incites in the human body a kind of illness peculiar to itself; one should apply in the disease to be healed . . . that remedy which is able to stimulate another artificially produced disease as similar as possible.' He had extended his generalisation from fevers, stating that this principle is applicable particularly in chronic diseases. As proof of these assertions he quoted a number of medicines tested.

We owe to Hahnemann this experimental approach, which marks the great advance in practical medicine. Others from Hippocrates down to Paracelsus had formulated the law of *similia similibus curentur*, but Paracelsus lacked the sure foundation of experiment on the healthy, and trusted almost entirely to a laborious and empirical testing of medicine on the sick.

The idea of the wholeness of man seems to have been lost by the medical classifiers and inventors of systems. Their classifications, while all-embracing and all-inclusive, covered everything about the illness they were describing but nothing about the patient himself. As an individual he was lost in the accumulation of detail. 'Man as an individual was being left to the philanthropist – the public-minded citizen.' Fortunately Hahnemann was not only a doctor but also a philanthropist.

Two years after his experiments with cinchona bark, he had undertaken the care of a mental patient of considerable fame. Once again he approached the problem *de novo* and departed from the treatment customary at that time. Indeed he appears to have anticipated the famous Pinel who, on his appointment to the Bicêtre Hospital in Paris in September 1793, decided at once to remove the chains and fetters from the mental patients there. It is interesting to note that Pinel too was violently opposed to blood-letting and the indiscriminate use of drugs.

In June 1792, the author Klockenburg was brought as a patient to Hahnemann. He spent the first few weeks in observation only, without giving any medical treatment. In reporting this case subsequently, Hahnemann wrote that he never allowed any insane person to be punished by blows or other painful bodily chastisement. 'The physician in charge of such unhappy people must have at his command an attitude which inspires respect but also creates confidence. He will never feel insulted by them. Their outbreaks of unreasonable anger only arouse his sympathy for their pitiful state and call forth his charity to relieve their sad condition.' The patient made a complete recovery and resumed his official position.

This study of an individual patient over several months, free from the preconceptions and prejudices of current teaching, is an illuminating example of Hahnemann's attitude to his patients. Again and again he laid stress on the importance of careful observation. The natural history of disease and its cure was his subject. He took care of the minutest details – *de minimis curet medicus* – and he had a genius for selecting the significant detail.

Three children in a large family had succumbed to a very bad attack of scarlet fever. 'The eldest daughter who had up to that time been taking Belladonna internally for some other external disease of the finger joints was the only one who refused to sicken with the fever, to my surprise . . . she was always the first to catch any other disease that happened to be prevalent.' Hahnemann followed up this clue at once. He gave Belladonna in very small doses to the remaining children of this numerous family and they all remained well, even though it was not possible to isolate them from their infected brothers and sisters.

Because he was concerned with details that might prove significant, Hahnemann had a great distrust of the 'lumpers'. If he had been a botanist he would have been a 'splitter'. He wrote, 'The theory of simplification has been the pet hobby of systematisers', and naturally therefore he had no use for Dr John Brown's theory that all patients could be classified into sthenics and asthenics, a theory that had a considerable vogue in Germany at the time.

Hahnemann had returned to Hippocratism – the enlightened medical empiricism which demands that the physician desists from speculation and limits himself to strict observations of the patient; that he follows each stage of the disease carefully until the very end . . . all signs of disease are important, as well as their succession and the time of their appearance and disappearance. A good understanding of the course of the disease is sometimes more important than a knowledge of its cause.

It was exactly on these principles that he conducted his experiments, or 'provings', using the word in its archaic sense of 'testing' – the exception *tests* the rule – on the action of medicines on healthy human beings. The course of the artificial illness was studied in the minutest detail, and the substitute patients were questioned and cross-questioned until the doctor was satisfied about the genuine nature of the symptoms.

He wrote to Dr Stapf, 'Whenever my provers present me with such a list I go through the symptoms with them, and question them right and left so as to complete from their recollection whatever requires to be more explicit, such as time, and the conditions under which the changes took place.'

These experiments demanded courage of a high order. For the sake of this research he risked his own health and that of his children, because he carried out the experiments not only on his collaborators but on himself and his family. At that time nobody knew what effects the poisons and medicines might have. Shortly after the publication of his first researches, a royal physician remonstrated with him, saying he must be undermining his health and that such experiments should only be conducted on criminals.

What was so remarkable was that Hahnemann not only had the vision to realise the necessity for the proving of medicines, but that he also combined with this wide power of conceptual thinking the genius to isolate the essence of the 'remedy' from the hundreds of symptoms recorded by himself and his collaborators. Many other doctors have carried out experimental provings, and indeed new remedies are still being tested on healthy human subjects according to his methods. It is doubtful if any physician has excelled Hahnemann in the clarity and penetration with which he isolated the distinctive features of the drug-illness. His powers of insight into the variety of differences and contrasts, and indeed the specific pattern of the symptoms produced, have never been equalled. Moreover, his experiences in this experimental pharmacology brought home to him not only the differences in the properties of the remedies, but also the differences between healthy individuals. He soon realised that for some of the weaker medicines, the provers must be individuals who were healthy but also of very irritable, delicate constitutions. He found that some individuals are affected by a very small quantity and that it was therefore wise to begin with the smallest dose. He learned that all the symptoms a medicine can produce are not observable in one person – so it must be tested on many to ascertain its full range of action.

Among the modifications produced by the tested remedy, Hahnemann attached great importance to alterations in the state of the disposition and mind of the prover. He regarded these changes as being of great significance, and in applying the results of his researches in the treatment of patients he claimed that the state of the disposition of the patient often chiefly determined the selection of the homoeopathic remedy.

For example, 'Aconite will seldom or never effect either a rapid or permanent cure in a patient of quiet, calm, equable disposition, and just as little will Nux Vomica be serviceable where the disposition is mild and phlegmatic, Pulsatilla where it is gay, happy and obstinate, or Ignatia where it is imperturbable.'

Hahnemann searched for the specific, not for the disease, but for the individual patient. This was one of the great contributions that he made to medicine. He taught physicians to respect the patient, to listen patiently and without interruption to the details of the history of his or her sufferings. A cure depended on this individualising examination of each case.

He maintained his standards to the end of his life, and at the age of eighty-two, when living in Paris, his first examination and investigation of a new patient lasted an hour and a half. One young patient recorded that he had to lie in bed and the doctor 'examined me more minutely than any doctor hitherto had done.'

Hahnemann was one of the great natural historians of disease and its cure. In his day, the little group of men who devoted their lives to what was then known as natural history were whole men confronting a whole world, not human beings floating in a culture medium.

Samuel Hahnemann certainly lived the life according to the truths that he discovered – and he certainly created the background in those tremendous compendiums of knowledge, the *Materia Medica Pura* and his *Chronic Diseases*. It was left for his followers to create the necessary institutions, the hospitals, the learned societies, the journals and the libraries.

Chapter 3

The Introduction of Homoeopathy into Great Britain

The introduction of homoeopathy into Great Britain was brought about by Hahnemann's first English disciple, Frederick Foster Hervey Quin. Quin was born in 1799, and his early history leaves many gaps. He once spoke of himself as being entirely alone for many years, a bachelor, no brother, no sister. The presumption must be that he was one of the children of the mist, which was the current euphemism of the great ladies of that time.

Perhaps his Christian names contain a clue. Frederick Foster was the name of the first husband of 'Dearest Bess', Lady Elizabeth Foster, the third party in the remarkable Devonshire House Triangle; she subsequently became the Duchess of Devonshire, and appointed Quin her travelling physician.

Another clue is his Christian name of Hervey, Lady Foster's maiden name, for she was the daughter of the famous Earl of Bristol, whose Grand Tours abroad have been commemorated by Hotel Bristols all over the continent of Europe.

At the age of sixteen, as soon as possible after the Battle of Waterloo, he went to Paris to study French. So successful a student was he that he was reputed to speak French better than English. He qualified as a doctor in Edinburgh in 1820, and almost at once was appointed by the British government as physician to the ex-Emperor Napoleon at St Helena. Evidently he had already made a deep impression as a young man of forceful character to be selected for such a post, but on the eve of his departure the news came of Napoleon's death.

Those were the days of great patrons and it was then that Quin was appointed physician to the Duchess of Devonshire. He appears to have made his first contact with homoeopathy in 1821 in Naples, where Dr de Romani, a homoeopathic doctor, was a physician to the Queen Maria Amalia of Naples. It was this same Dr de Romani who converted the Comte de Guidi, a French doctor, to homoeopathic practice and so was responsible for the introduction of homoeopathy to France.

Quin had been ill himself, and had been purged and sweated, blistered and bled. In one illness five pints of his blood were removed. When he was next taken ill, so seriously that his life was despaired of, instead of the usual blistering and bleeding he was given only five small powders which had no taste other than that of sugar, and he recovered.

When the Duchess of Devonshire died in 1824, Quin was appointed physician to Prince Leopold of Saxe-Coburg, the famous Uncle Leopold of Queen Victoria's letters. And in attendance on the Prince, Quin travelled about Europe and once again visited Italy. At that time all the published work on homoeopathy was in German. In Rome he met Dr Necher, who had accompanied the Austrian army to Italy; impressed once again with the successes of homoeopathic medicine he learned German, in order to read and study the methods, and went to visit Hahnemann at Koethen. He maintained his friendship with Hahnemann throughout his life.

In the following year, 1827, he came with Prince Leopold to London where, with his numerous connections with the aristocracy, he introduced homoeopathy among the upper ranks of society. He was well qualified to do this, for he was a man of charming good manners. He was a wonderful storyteller and soon became a welcome guest at the tables of some of the highest personages in the land. The Prince of Wales (afterwards King Edward VIII) regarded Quin as a dear friend; he was on intimate terms with Charles Dickens, Sir Edwin Landseer and a host of famous artists and actors. In England at that time the names of Hahnemann and homoeopathy were unknown and his patients were dubbed 'Quinnites'.

Four years later in Austria-Hungary a severe epidemic of Asiatic cholera broke out. This was an opportunity to test the principles of homoeopathy and Quin went out to Brünn in Moravia to relieve the homoeopathic doctor, who had himself fallen ill. Quin also contracted cholera but recovered under homoeopathic treatment. The doctor to whose aid he went treated 681 cases with a mortality of less than 5%, while at the same time in other hands the mortality was 50% in cases treated on orthodox lines. When he returned to England he published an account of his experiences and this time settled in London for good.

Quin was well aware of the opposition that homoeopathy was likely to encounter from the medical profession. His visits to Hahnemann and his numerous European contacts kept him informed of the difficulties the new system was encountering all over Europe. The Czar of Russia, impressed by the results of homoeopathic treatment in an epidemic of trachoma in the Cadet School at St Petersburg, resolved to introduce homoeopathic treatment into the army medical service. But even against the will of such an autocrat the Russian doctors were successful in intro- ducing regulations which made the practice of homoeopathy almost impossible. Quin knew, too, that homoeopathy had been forbidden in Austria by an Imperial Edict inspired by the Court physicians, and he realised that if homoeopathy were to succeed in England, it was essential to avoid antagonising the medical profession. From his own contacts with Hahnemann he must have felt that if the Master had been more of a man of the world, homoeopathy would not have been presented in such sharp contrast and in such violent antagonism to the old system of medicine.

He was therefore not long in drawing up a code of conduct for homoeopathic practitioners, and this was drafted by 1834. Two years later the Censor of the Royal College of Physicians sent Quin a warning notice, which he ignored. It was after this that some of his friends nominated him for election to the Athenaeum Club, but before the election a Dr Paris, a member of the club, saw the nomination on the notice board and protested with many slanderous accusations that no homoeopath should be elected. Dr Paris had been the Censor whose warning notice Quin had ignored. Paris was a lecturer in materia medica and had made 5000 guineas by the sale of his textbook, which was the current standard work of therapeutics. On election night this physician arrived with forty colleagues from a meeting at the Royal College of Physicians and the result was forty-four blackballs against Quin's election, a record for the club! Quin felt that the language indulged in by this physician could not be allowed to pass without impunity and challenged him to a duel, but his opponent climbed down with an ample apology.

Quin was anxious to give his orthodox colleagues no grounds for complaint against medical etiquette. He never attempted to answer any attack on himself in the newspapers or medical journals. For several years he refused fees for medical advice, so that no interested or personal motives could be attributed to him. He also published his scientific writings in French or Latin, so that he could not be accused of writing popular books. He even dedicated a translation of one of Hahnemann's books to the President of the Royal College of Physicians – taking the bull by the horns with a vengeance.

But 'this quiet mole-like burrowing', as one of his colleagues termed it, was not understood by his colleagues and still less by interested laymen. Hahnemann, now practising in Paris, had several English patients who actually went over to France for consultations. Among the more energetic of them was the Reverend Everest of Wickwar who, in

1834, was the first to write in English on homoeopathy and published a pamphlet of forty pages addressed to the medical practitioners of Great Britain.

Another energetic patient was William Leaf, one of the most wealthy merchants of the City of London. He had been completely cured of a chronic disease by Hahnemann and adopted the cause of homoeopathy with great vigour. Leaf demanded of Quin that he should make the teachings of Hahnemann better known by the publication of popular writings, but Quin could not agree. Undeterred, Mr Leaf went over to Paris and brought back with him Dr Curie, grandfather of the husband of the famous Madame Curie.

Leaf financed a small hospital where Dr Curie gave clinical demonstrations, and backed numerous popular publications on homoeopathy compiled in English by Curie. Leaf also organised a dispensary for the poor, where Dr Curie treated numerous patients every Sunday. Thus the homoeopathic physicians were divided on the question of appealing to the public. Quin was convinced that the homoeopathic physicians could only continue practice by keeping within the bounds of professional etiquette, but these rules were too much for the ardour of his younger colleagues. It is perhaps not surprising that when Quin called a meeting of the five homoeopathic doctors at the time of Queen Victoria's accession, no agreement could be reached on the rules of his projected Homoeopathic Society.

But if Quin at that date was a prophet without honour in his own country, in France he was highly esteemed. Hahnemann had been made Life President of Honour of the French Homoeopathic Society and automatically took the chair at any meeting at which he was present. When Hahnemann died in 1843 this signal honour was accorded to Quin as Hahnemann's greatest successor.

The following year, on the 10th April 1844, the anniversary of Hahnemann's birthday, a little band of eight devoted men sat around a baize-covered table in Quin's house. Fifty years later the sole survivor, Dr Cameron, described the scene. Presiding was Quin, an imposing figure, with high-domed forehead, bald except for tufts of curly hair over his ears, level eyebrows, a piercing glance, a strong chiselled nose, a long upper lip, a firm lower lip, a broad chin, hollow cheeks framed by mutton-chop whiskers. A silk-faced frockcoat, a light double-breasted waistcoat and a striped silk stock indicated not so much the correct professional attire of the day, but the fashion of an age that passed away with Count d'Orsay.

Quin was fond of having his own way and this time he succeeded in

17

gaining the assent of his colleagues to the laws he had drafted. Law 121 of the society read that the President of the Society shall not be allowed to resign his office without the consent of two-thirds of the society, and while Quin lived he was never allowed to resign – a presidency of 34 years! Before he died, the tiny society of eight had reached a membership of 292.

But Quin's labours were not ended. A scientific journal was started, as the laws of the society forbade members to communicate results of treatment to lay journals. A library was founded and Quin concerned himself with the foundation of the London Homoeopathic Hospital, initially in Golden Square.

In 1854, the year of the Crimean War, homoeopathy came through its first great test in England with flying colours. That year London suffered a severe epidemic of cholera. The President of the Board of Health appointed a Medical Council to collect statistics showing the results of treatment of the epidemic. The Council collected returns from all the London hospitals, including the London Homoeopathic Hospital. The returns from the Homoeopathic Hospital were vastly superior to those of other hospitals. Was it significant that the figures from this hospital were suppressed by the Council in their report presented to Parliament? Lord Ebury, a governor of the hospital and Member of Parliament for Middlesex, obtained a copy of the suppressed report from the London Homoeopathic Hospital and this was presented to Parliament as a special Parliamentary paper.

Perhaps this successful demonstration of the value of homoeopathic practice stimulated a reaction from the orthodox profession. At any rate, three years later an Act to regulate the Qualifications of Practitioners in Medicine and Surgery was passing through Parliament. It was on the point of being read for the third time in the House of Lords when it was discovered that it afforded no protection against the rejection of candidates for degrees and diplomas if they were suspected of homoeopathic leanings.

This was no idle fear, as a candidate had been rejected by the Edinburgh faculty on account of his homoeopathic beliefs; a graduate of St Andrews was commanded to return his diploma; and a candidate in Aberdeen was refused permission to pass his last examination because he declined to sign a written declaration pledging himself never to practise homoeopathy. Quin and others sought Lord Ebury's aid and a clause was drawn up for insertion in the Bill which protected future candidates. Lord Ebury succeeded in introducing this new clause, the Charter of the Rights of Homoeopathy, on the third reading.

This political success did not endear Quin to his orthodox colleagues. It is not surprising that the President of the College of Physicians refused to meet him, even when requested to do so by Queen Victoria, to discuss Disraeli's serious illness.

Quin's last signature in the Minute Book of the Homoeopathic Society is dated 1866, but he lived another twelve years in partial retirement before he died in 1878. He left the bulk of his fortune to the London Homoeopathic Hospital.

I have described at some length the career of the first British homoeopathic physician, because I would like the reader to have some insight into the difficulties that he had to overcome, and to remind him of the strictly professional code to which he always adhered.

Homoeopathy in Bristol
In 1843 a retired Naval surgeon, Mr Trotman of Park Street, was to be found in the Bristol Directory describing himself as a surgeon-homoeopathist. In the previous year the Directory adds at the end of the list of Physicians and Surgeons the name of a Mr Stock, a 'professed cupper', but in 1844 his name disappears from the list. Had Mr Trotman put him out of business? Mr Trotman had studied under Hahnemann in Paris and five years later was joined by Dr Black, an energetic Scot from Edinburgh, a former President of the Hunterian Medical Society, who had already made his mark as a homoeopathic physician. He was bursting with ideas, a tremendous organiser and a great debater. He had started a homoeopathic dispensary in Edinburgh with his friend and co-editor, Dr Russell. He organised the first Homoeopathic Congress in Cheltenham in 1850, was Chairman of the 2nd Congress in London in the following year, and four years after his arrival in Bristol opened the first homoeopathic dispensary in that city, in 1852, with another Scot as the resident surgeon.

In the following year two more homoeopathic physicians arrived and from that date onwards there seem to have been never less than four homoeopathic physicians practising in Clifton and Bristol. The dispensaries moved about from one street to another, sometimes being conducted from the doctor's own residence.

One of the most remarkable of the early Bristol homoeopaths was Dr Eubulus Williams, one-time Surgeon to the 1st Gloucestershire Volunteers and senior surgeon to the Bristol Hospital for Sick Children. Convinced of the principles of homoeopathy, in 1867 he felt it his duty to his hospital committee and subscribers to announce his change of views in a printed address, leaving it with them to decide whether they still desired to retain his services. Subsequently he was appointed Physician to Muller's Orphanage, and in 1873 had to deal with an epidemic of smallpox which was ravaging that institution. He published the results of a series of ninety cases without a death and with minimal scarring of the face.

It was in 1883 that through the generosity of two Clifton ladies the Homoeopathic Hospital was founded in Brunswick Square, and in 1903 wards were opened for in-patients. In 1917 Mr Melville Wills promised to build a new hospital at Cotham House as a memorial to his son, Captain Bruce Wills, who was killed in 1915. The foundation stone was laid in 1921 by H.R.H. the Prince of Wales, and the hospital was opened in 1925 by H.R.H. Princess Helena Victoria.

Chapter 4

The Quest for Specifics

In the very earliest ages of medicine, the main objective of the legendary physicians was the discovery of specifics. Aesculapius himself was famous because of his knowledge of specifics, and the votive tablets hung in his temples were records of specific cures. The marvellous remedy was the 'arcanum', a secret of the alchemists. Bacon, in *The Advancement of Learning*, deplored the lack of specific medicines and quoted the then current jest that English physicians were like bishops that had the keys of binding and loosing but no more. The philosopher Locke commented: 'Did we know the mechanical affections of the particles of rhubarb, hemlock, opium and of a man as a watchmaker does that of a watch, we would be able to tell that rhubarb will purge, hemlock kill, and opium make a man sleep.'

Sydenham claimed that a specific was a medicine – not a palliative – that cured a disease; and the only true specific that he recognised was the Peruvian bark for intermittent fever. It is worthy of note that this was the medicine Hahnemann tested; a true specific in his search for its principle of action and thus the inductive route to his reasoning-out of the principle of the simillimum. In his *similia similibus curentur*, Hahnemann had uncovered the principle on which specifics could be found, and for the next six years he proved drug after drug, one specific after another.

Cullen's *Materia Medica* was not the only textbook he translated in the last decade of the 18th century. There was also Munro's textbook, a thesaurus by a London MRCP and von Haller's *Materia Medica*. Hahnemann was critical of the claims of these physicians for so-called specifics against undifferentiated groups of disorders; he wrote that grand plans were formed by medical men for discovering nothing less than a universal specific for everything they called poison; and this included the plague, philtres, bewitchment and the bites of venomous animals. Among other agents this specific was sought for in vinegar. Hahnemann condemned a qualified doctor who advertised aspirin for the toothache as certain to cure. He commented: 'that toothache is as various in character as are the internal maladies that produce it; hence one medicine is useful only in one kind, and another in another kind of toothache.'

He gives three examples of different kinds of toothache and their three appropriate remedies, remedies which are not palliatives but permanently curative. Of course, to begin with there was inevitably a hangover from his early training; he found some difficulty in giving up concepts of diseases as entities in themselves; so he began by searching for specifics for different diseases, such as mercury for syphilis and thuja for gonorrhoea. But he was soon disillusioned with the 'named diseases' of orthodox medicine; he found that they were not of a constant character and did not conform to a fixed form. Indeed, that the name of a disease was in itself an imaginary thing to be cured, and that the few true specifics had been discovered by accident, specifics for the few illnesses which always preserved the same character. But why no more than these few specifics? . . . 'Because all other diseases only present themselves as individual cases of disease differing from each other, or as epidemics which have never been seen before, and will never be seen again in exactly the same form.' What foresight. No high-powered microscopes, no bacteriology, no virus experts in his day.

In 1792 he was rather pessimistic about epidemics and admitted that 'we know of no specific antidotes for the several kinds of contagious matters; we must content ourselves with general prophylactic means.' Six years later, however, he reported on an epidemic of influenza in which the remedy Camphor surpassed all his expectations. He claimed that it was a specific in all stages of the disease, especially when it was given as early as possible and in large doses. A large number of patients recovered in four days in spite of their serious symptoms. In the next year, 1799, an epidemic of scarlet fever reached the town where he was living. Faced with an early case in a child of ten, he recalled that Belladonna was the remedy capable of producing a counterpart of the little girl's symptoms and prescribed a dose in the 6x potency. The child recovered on the second day; he then prescribed Belladonna for the other five children in the family and they all remained perfectly well.

By 1809 Germany, and indeed much of Europe, was suffering from a feverish epidemic which was being treated, very unsuccessfully, as if it were a malarial infection. Hahnemann described the symptoms in detail when they had not been altered by drugs, and matched these with his description in Latin of the symptoms of the toxicology of Nux Vomica in his *Fragmenta de Viribus Medicamentorium Positivis*, which he had published four years before, in 1805. He found Nux Vomica the only medicine capable of curing a great proportion of the infected patients in a short time. He had to admit that in some severe cases there were patients whose symptoms were not covered by Nux Vomica, and that these states were matched by the symptoms produced by Arsenic, a mineral which had fallen out of favour with orthodox physicians as too dangerous in ordinary doses, but which Hahnemann found efficacious when given in the 12x potency.

For the typhus epidemic of 1812 he recommended one drop of Bryonia in the morning, and if no improvement by the fourth day, a single drop of Rhus Tox. 12c. But if in spite of this a comatose state developed, he recommended a dose of very dilute sweet spirit of nitre every six hours. It was natural that even his most devoted followers should find it difficult to accept these recommendations. His favourite pupil, Stapf, whose daughter the great chief had been treating by correspondence, received a letter from him with the accusation: 'The frequently repeated doses of Spongia, although small, became in your daughter's case a wrong and therefore injurious medicine on account of the repetition.'

In 1821, an epidemic mistakenly diagnosed by the profession as scarlet fever appeared, which Hahnemann distinguished as purpura miliaris; this often proved fatal in orthodox hands. He recommended Aconite 10x, a single dose to be followed in 16–24 hours by Coffea 6x. He added: 'Nothing should be done or given to the patient – no venesection, no leeches, no calomel, no purgatives, no cooling or diaphor-medicines or herb tea, no water compresses, no baths, no clysters, no gargles, no vesicatories (blisters) or sinapisms (mustard plasters).'

Cholera invaded Europe in 1831. Hahnemann tackled the problem energetically and published four pamphlets free of charge. His advice proved very valuable. The Hungarian Dr Bakody had 154 cholera patients from the end of July to the beginning of September; only 6 died. This compared with 122 deaths out of 284 hospital patients and 699 deaths out of 1217 cholera patients treated privately in the same town.

A Prussian Medical Officer of Health wrote in July to Hahnemann asking him to suggest a specific remedy because a Russian ship had docked at Danzig only fifteen miles away, and already five hundred Danzigers had died. How did Hahnemann, who had not seen or treated a single cholera patient, find the remedy with such complete conviction?

He explained that he procured from some careful observers a very accurate description of the commencing symptoms, and found that the first and most important symptoms of the patients were like the symptoms produced by a healthy individual who had taken a large dose of camphor. Camphor, therefore, should be the best remedy to be given at the onset of the infection, according to his law of similars. He insisted on the very early recognition of the disease; only in the first two hours of the sickness would Camphor abort the infection. If the disease had advanced to the second and third stages, he advised the use of Cuprum and/or Veratrum Album.

In an influenza epidemic in Bristol in 1939 I found that Gelsemium was the most frequently used remedy; but I did not find that Gelsemium covered the hospital admissions of influenza that were complicated by pneumonia. Of the persons who contract complications, I am of the opinion that these patients are constitutionally different from the general run and are likely to require a different remedy. In my ward, I had five patients with influenzal pneumonia at the same time, and as far as I can remember they all required different remedies.

Another exception to the general response to the epidemic remedy is the patient who has undergone a recent inoculation. Soon after the blitzes began in Bristol, a huge shelter population began to gather each night, and as a protective measure it was decided to inoculate the nursing staff at the hospital against diphtheria and typhoid. Two months later, the hospital was smitten with a mild influenzal type of infection and about a dozen nurses went sick in a couple of days. They were typically Bryonia, and the nurses cleared up promptly in forty-eight hours, all except one who had been recently inoculated; her temperature failed to come down, all her sinuses were infected and until she had a dose of Morbillinum she made no improvement.

Perhaps it is in children that the best results from the epidemic remedy can still be expected, for they have not been exposed to so many decades of antibiotics. The increased resistance of infecting agents to antibiotics is well known. It should also be understood that the repeated use of antibiotics inhibits the patient's immune system and thus his natural healing capacity. In these circumstances a homoeopathic remedy may not produce as great an effect as could otherwise be expected.

In some homoeopathic circles the specific remedy is used in low potency. Quite early on in my practice I realised that the choice of remedy, whatever the circumstances, was to be based on the totality of the symptoms – that is, the mental and general, as well as the particular symptoms of the patient – whichever potency was chosen.

It has also been said that the lowest potencies only influence those regions where local tissue changes have occurred, and that they have no influence on the mental and general symptoms of the patient. However, in my experience low potencies certainly do influence the whole patient, and for this reason too I have had to conclude that our choice of remedy should be based on the totality of symptoms and not on tissue change alone.

Apart from the epistemology, what do we learn from this review? Firstly, that in comparison with the four specifics known to Hahnemann before his provings, there is a range of specifics for the infectious diseases and for tissue disorders.

These specifics are important in teaching homoeopathy. Any enquiry into the way in which orthodox practitioners are convinced of the value of homoeopathic prescribing demonstrates that the great majority are profoundly impressed by the personal experience of a rapid cure of an acute illness, either in themselves or in one of their patients, when they themselves have failed.

Secondly, that the teaching of homoeopathy should not only be theoretical but must also include practical experience. What more certain confirmation is available than the demonstration to the doctor in his own practice of the value of specifics?

Chapter 5

Constitutional Prescribing

In the late 1940s I was asked by the National Association of Mental Health to carry out research into the social adaptation of children brought up in institutions and orphanages. The hypothesis was that these children, deprived of normal home life and brought up in communities of children, were less likely to be successful in adapting to the working world when the time came to leave school. In short, that the environment of the orphanage and the poor-law home lacked essential factors required for normal maturity.

It was possible to demonstrate that orphanage children were at some disadvantage, but what emerged from the survey was that these children were as much handicapped by inherited constitutional factors as by their upbringing. This finding was against the stream of current psychiatric thought and invoked considerable criticism in some quarters. And not surprisingly, for while the child-guidance experts were skilled at manipulating the environment to suit the child's needs, they were pessimistic about their capacity to alter radically the child's inborn temperament.

My experience as a homoeopath to some extent contradicted the official pessimism. In other fields of medicine than child psychiatry, I considered that it had been possible to modify temperaments and influence constitutional factors. I do not claim for homoeopathic remedies that they can alter cerebral dominance, change a left-handed child to a right-handed child, or restore pigment to an albino. However, I think most of us will agree that we expect to improve 'sustained tolerance' to stress and improve 'affective regulation'. In other words, we expect our remedies to help patients to bear with the slings and arrows of outrageous fortune and to assist them to maintain a normal emotional balance.

How far are we justified in these beliefs? Theoretically, this is the only field for homoeopathic medicine in the treatment of the neurotic child. Are these beliefs in the power of medicines derived from the use of herbal medicines? Nicholas Culpeper, writing of motherwort, said,

'There is no better herb to take melancholy vapours from the heart, to strengthen it, and make a merry, cheerful, blithe soul.' But Culpeper's system of medicine was based on the astrological premises of the influence of the stars, and assumed that the therapeutic effect of plants was controlled by the stars. Participation was assumed. Of *Viscum* he states: '(You) can also take for granted that that which grows upon oaks, participates something of the nature of Jupiter, because the oak is one of his trees.'

And if *Viscum* was under Jupiter, *Digitalis* was under Venus, *Hyoscyamus* under Saturn, *Hypericum* under the sun, *Bryonia* under Mars, and *Dulcamara* under Mercury. It was Hahnemann who liberated us from a pharmacology based on the participation mystique so essential in the thinking of primitive man and children.

There are times when I find some confusion in Hahnemann's writing. (This may be the effect of translation from one language to another.) I find a tendency in places for Hahnemann to rank the disposition of the patient as a symptom, and it is not always clear whether he means by this the disposition of the patient when in normal health, or the alterations in disposition produced by disease. For example, he writes: 'This holds good to such an extent, that the state of the disposition of the patient often chiefly determines the selection of the homoeopathic remedy, as being a decidedly characteristic symptom.'

Scattered through the *Materia Medica* and his *Chronic Diseases* are observations, based, it must be inferred, on clinical experience rather than provings. For example, of Phosphorus he comments, before listing the symptoms recorded by the provers, that 'it will rarely be found appropriate where lack of sexual impulse and weakness in the genital parts is manifest.' Which I take to mean that he recommends Phosphorus only in patients with highly-sexed temperaments. Or of Capsicum: 'Diseases curable by Capsicum are rarely met with in persons of tense fibre'. Or of Chamomilla: 'It is unsuited for persons who bear pain calmly and patiently.' He adds, 'I attach great importance to this observation.'

We are apt to take our modern remedy pictures for granted. In practice, our present concept of many remedies has been built up on the foundations of the provings by more than a century's clinical experience. However, I think it is important to make a distinction between the alterations in the mood brought about by the remedy provings, and the disposition most suited to a particular remedy, which may not necessarily have been indicated by provings.

This involves some research in our original sources, and I have compared Hahnemann's reports of provings in the *Materia Medica Pura* and the *Chronic Diseases* with Hering's collection of cured symptoms in *Guiding Symptoms*. It is not always clear, even in Hahnemann's lists of symptoms, how far they were derived from actual provings and how far they were observations made on patients under treatment. By limiting oneself to the symptoms that are followed by a note of the time interval, one can be fairly sure that one is dealing with actual provings. Take, for example, Chamomilla. All but thirty of the four hundred and ninety-odd symptoms are Hahnemann's own observations. Of the mental symptoms recorded with time intervals, these occur:

Dullness of senses.

Piteous moaning because he cannot have what he wants.

Whining restlessness; the child wants this and that, which when offered is refused or pushed away.

Cannot endure being spoken to, or interrupted when speaking.

She seeks a cause for being peevish at everything.

She cannot return a civil answer.

Easily chagrined and excited to anger.

Excessive uneasiness, anxiety, agonised tossing about.

All these symptoms are marked by Hering with the sign signifying 'repeatedly verified by cures'. The evidence therefore supports the hypothesis that Chamomilla can produce an alteration in mood.

Investigations and comparisons of provings and cured symptoms confirm that alterations in mood can be brought about by Hepar Sulph., Argentum Nit. (using the provings recorded in Allen's *Handbook of the Materia Medica*), Arsenicum Album and Capsicum.

It would be a useful exercise to make these comparisons between what we classify as mental symptoms in the provings and the records of cured symptoms for many more of our remedies. Subsequent experience confirms Hahnemann's claims that potentised remedies can alter moods, and even dispositions. In one of his dramatic footnotes he comments, 'How often do we not meet with a mild, soft disposition in patients who have for years been afflicted with the most painful diseases, so that the physician feels constrained to esteem and have compassion on the sufferer? But if he subdue the disease and restore the patient to health – he is often astonished and horrified at the frightful alteration in his disposition. He often witnesses the occurrence of ingratitude, cruelty, refined malice and propensities most disgraceful and degrading to humanity.'

Chapter 6

General Psychiatry

Hahnemann stated in *The Organon* that 'The organism is indeed the material instrument of life, but it is not conceivable without the animation imparted to it by the instinctively perceiving *dynamis*, just as the "vital force" is not conceivable without the organism; consequently the two together constitute a unity, although in thought our mind separates this unity into two distinct concepts for the sake of easy comprehension.' (*Organon*, 6th Edition, trans., Philadelphia, 1922, Paragraph 15.)*

Hahnemann would quite probably have agreed with the modern psychiatric view that perceives the individual as of body and mind, two incomplete entities uniting to form a whole. Disease is a condition of matter – the body – but matter can have an influence on the mind, as in the organic dementias such as general paralysis of the insane, encephalitis lethargica, and the effects of leucotomy. It is also possible to conceive of disease or alienation of the mind without any disease of the body – the endogenous psychoses.

On the other hand, this postulate is rejected by other psychiatrists as imaginary. The psychoses, they say, are somatoses. In the psychoses the personality no longer functions as a governor and a mechanism subject to organic laws takes over. The pilot has fainted; the automatic pilot takes over. Dr Kretschmer claims no sharp division between organic and psychogenic illnesses. He draws attention to the fact that the modern tendency is to treat psychoses by physical methods and to treat bodily disorders such as asthma and eczema by psychotherapy. It was the Italian Baglive, a seventeenth-century pathologist, who coined the aphorism 'The patient is the doctor's best textbook.' Psychiatrists were slow to learn that therapy itself discovered new facts and was indeed an instrument of research.

What can we learn from the homoeopathic treatment of the psy-

*All subsequent paragraph references are taken from this edition of *The Organon*.

choses? When the psychoses are arranged in their order of response to homoeopathic treatment one finds a certain pattern. The psychoses most accessible to homoeopathic treatment, in my opinion, are the confusional states, the deliria of infectious disorders, of cardiac failure and anaemia. Hahnemann speaks of severe somatic diseases, bronchiectasis, puerperal sepsis, where the illness becomes transformed into an insanity, a kind of melancholia or mild mania (Paragraph 216). One thinks of Bryonia in pneumococcal infections, of Baptisia in typhoid infections and Weil's disease, of Laurocerasus in cardiac deliriums and of Cannabis Indica in uraemia. In all these conditions there is a large somatic component – a septicaemia, a defective cerebral circulation with a consequent relative anoxia, a direct toxic effect on the neurones.

The next psychosis most easily influenced by homoeopathic treatment is involutional melancholia. Though associated with a definite body type, there is no evidence of heredity. It appears to be a post-climacteric phenomenon of a biochemical basis, and responds to such remedies as Aurum, Selenium and Sepia.

When we come to the next group of major mental illnesses – the manic depressive psychoses – we are confronted with conditions that are much more difficult to modify.* There are few such patients that reach me who have not had electroconvulsive therapy, and the picture is thereby complicated by what resembles a post-concussion syndrome. Very often this must be tackled first. I have had little response from Arnica, but quite good results after Natrum Sulph.

In assessing the results of treatment in manic depressive psychosis we must always take into consideration the tendency to spontaneous cure. It is possible to see the patient for the first time at the end of a depressive cycle. A prescription is given and the patient reports a marvellous improvement and yet, when months or years later the next depressive cycle arrives, the same prescription has no influence. The recovery was spontaneous and not attributable to the remedy. Even though it is possible to help many of these patients in the depressed phase – to relieve them of some of their depression, and support them sufficiently to enable them to hold down their jobs or housekeep for their families, with such remedies as Kali Carb. and Lachesis – I have never convinced myself that I have made a radical impression on the depressive process.

Examples can be given. A young schoolteacher, who had given up her job, wept continually and could only get through one day at a time. Under treatment with Kali Carb. she can look forward to her marriage in

*Dr Bodman wrote this material before the advent of the anti-depressant drugs.

a year's time and has begun to buy furniture for her home, although she is still not well enough to teach a class of forty five-year-olds. Another patient, a married woman who was suicidal when brought to me, sat about in her house doing nothing. She describes herself as still confused, still in a muddle at home, but she does not panic when there are a great many things to be done. The incredible muddle at home no longer worries her. She was a Lycopodium case. Another married woman, wife of a professional cricketer and whose depression was interfering seriously with his career – though still tearful at times, and still nervous of being alone (as so many potential suicides are), was able to let her husband go off to play for his county with the help of Causticum.

In patients with a short cycle of depression, recurring every few months, I have never been able to postpone the expected onset of the depression. (Incidentally, neither does electroconvulsive therapy alter the individual cycle.) I have been able to maintain very intelligent patients at their posts as university lecturers, but have never relieved them sufficiently to enable them to continue with their research or other creative work.

Hahnemann wrote of insanity or mania caused by fright, vexation and the abuse of alcohol. The mania would have broken out as an acute disease but in his view it almost always arises from internal psora. He says it must not be treated with antipsorics in the acute phase but with remedies such as Aconite, Belladonna, Stramonium, Hyoscyamus or Mercury (Paragraph 221). He observes later that if no anti-psoric treatment is exhibited during the remission, then the psora develops completely and passes into either a periodic or continued mental derangement, which is then more difficult to be cured by anti-psorics (Paragraph 223). It is clear from this that Hahnemann was familiar with manic-depressive psychosis although he ranks it as a somatic illness. Of course, 'la folie circulaire', as it was first called, was not recognised as a separate type of mental disease until 1854, after Hahnemann's death. It would certainly be worth while following up the experience of the Australian psychiatrists who have used lithium salts to control hypo-manic states, and I suggest that homoeopathic potencies of lithium salts might be of value in depression. The modern accidental provings of lithium make a fascinating story but would be too long a digression here.

The next psychosis to be considered in our graded scheme is schizo-phrenia. Here again there are difficulties in assessing the results of any treatment. There is a tendency to spontaneous remission. I have seen two remarkable recoveries in children, which in my view were not due to my prescribing, but may have been due to dramatic changes in their environment. Once again, here is a major mental illness with a specific hereditary factor. The pathology is obscure but possibly depends on a biochemical perversion at the level of the thalamus. Apart from the difficulties of securing the patient's cooperation in providing a full symptomatology, and his consent to taking any medicine at all, I can report very little success in curing these cases. I have relieved several patients by treating them with such remedies as Arsenicum Album for the fear and horror that their mental breakdown had aroused in themselves, but the underlying psychosis remained unchanged.

I had one university student who was studying social science and who in the course of her work became quite obsessed by the sexual deviations in the families she had to visit. These stories and the fantasies she built round them so completely preoccupied her mind that she had to give up her studies. She relapsed into a silly giggling state, continually asking questions which on the surface seemed irrelevant but which proved to be connected with her fantasies about the sex life of her clients. She was much relieved by Platina: the anxiety and preoccupations were much less intense, although the problems, she said, were still in her mind. However, they did not obtrude themselves and she was able to settle down to a somewhat routine domestic existence, though it was clear she was an unsuitable person to continue with such studies.

I found that other patients had a temporary increase in self-confidence and were more energetic and active after Silica, but the improvement was only temporary. An ex-soldier who had been demobilised after arduous service in Malaya had difficulty in settling down again at his father's farm. His father had an oesophageal stricture and the son could not bear to watch him at meal times. He became morose and silent, and one day smashed up the furniture in his room and tried to burn it. He no longer went to the pub for a drink at nights as he believed that people were talking about him. He was becoming more and more suspicious and the family doctor wanted to certify him, but after Silica he became more trustful and I persuaded him to farm in a different county. He is still very reserved and jerky in speech and action, but is holding down a job.

A Brazilian psychiatrist, Dr Buscaino, has pointed out the similarity of the effects of certain alkaloids on man to the schizophrenic picture – notably mescaline and opuntia cylindrica. Impressed by these resemblances, Buscaino considers that the primary lesion is due to toxic amines which fail to be destroyed by the reticulo-endothelial system and produce disseminated lesions in the cortex. He recommends treatment with T.A.B. vaccine to mobilise the defences of the organism – in effect a non-specific treatment with nosodes.

Once more Hahnemann appears to have noted the schizophrenic. Surely this is the illness he refers to in his reference to the chattering fool (the hebephrenic). This was one of the real mental maladies that he described, as opposed to those mental illnesses due to environmental stresses – which he lists as faults of education, bad practices, corrupt morals, neglect of the mind, superstition or ignorance (Paragraph 224). He claims these mental diseases of long standing sprang from somatic maladies, or else developed simultaneously with them (Paragraph 230).

Last on my list of major mental illnesses is paranoia. Here is an example of a purely psychological disturbance with no pathology and no somatic accompaniments. Again there is evidence of hereditary factors. These patients usually find their way into mental hospitals, although I followed one case as a private patient for three years. He had a classical Lachesis symptomatology – but there was no response to any potency even after intercurrent nosodes.

To summarise these findings, it would appear that the greater the somatic element in the psychosis, the better the response to homoeopathic treatment; but if the somatic element is minimal, and the psychological factor preponderant, the smaller the response to homoeopathic potencies. Such conclusions are no doubt surprising to the homoeopath who has learned to value the 'mental' symptoms in individualising his patient. But let me state Hahnemann's views on mental diseases. He writes, 'What are termed mental diseases do not constitute a class of disease sharply separated from the others, since in the so-called corporeal (or what we now call somatic) diseases the condition of the disposition and the mind is always altered, and in all cases of disease the state of the patient's disposition is to be particularly noted along with the totality of the symptoms.' (Paragraph 215). 'Almost all the so-called mental and emotional diseases are nothing more than corporeal (i.e. somatic) diseases, in which the symptoms of derangement of the mind and disposition peculiar to each is increased, while the somatic symptoms decline.' (Paragraph 215). Here Hahnemann's thinking is characteristic of his era. The terms 'natural philosopher' and 'nature' seem to have acquired an unconscious meaning of this earth. The word 'natural' seemed to have only the meaning of corporeal (somatic) existence. And indeed, in the *Dictionary of Psychological Medicine* published in 1892 by Dr Tuke, one of the most scientific and advanced psychiatrists of his day, insanity is defined as a brain disease.

We constantly refer to the totality of the symptoms; however, this does not necessarily mean the totality of the personality, but rather only the totality of the disease. Hahnemann began by stating: 'The sum of all the symptoms and conditions must be the sole indication – the sole guide to the remedy.' (Paragraph 18). But a little later he allows a slight modification: 'the greatest number of symptoms similar', expanding this concession in a footnote (to Paragraph 57): 'If only the stronger well-marked characteristic and peculiar symptoms of the disease are matched and covered by the same medicine with similarity of symptoms, the few opposite symptoms will disappear.' However, he blurs this clear-cut totality of the symptoms by introducing the concept of the disposition of the patient as an additional indication (Paragraph 210), and does this precisely in the field of mental diseases. He goes so far as to say: 'The state of disposition of the patient often chiefly determines the selection of the remedy, as being a decidedly characteristic symptom.' (Paragraph 211). The corollary follows in the next paragraph: 'No powerful medicinal substance in the world does not very notably alter the state of the disposition and mind in the healthy individual.' (Paragraph 212). Does a study of provings really substantiate this claim? Hahnemann's dispositions appear to represent emotional attitudes rather than intellectual qualities. He speaks of dispositions as soft, patient, chaste, modest, ungrateful, cruel, malicious, obstinate, violent, hasty, intolerant, capricious, impatient, desponding, lascivious and shameless. (Footnote 121).

I must admit that I find some confusion here and have difficulty in accepting a disposition or emotional attitude as a symptom pure and simple. I can say my leg is numb or my head aches, but *I* feel angry or bewildered. Are not symptoms referable to organs, and dispositions to the whole person? This opens up wide fields for discussion, such as the nature of personality and the interaction of body and mind. Without attempting to answer these questions, I would like to draw attention to some German theories of stratification of the personality. This of course is not a new idea. The American novelist Herman Melville in his last short story, *Billy Budd* (1888), speaks of the Captain 'letting himself melt back into what remains primeval in our formalised humanity'. These theories postulate the 'depth person' of early infancy 'living out of the old brain', seeking only to satisfy vital needs; but as the cerebral cortex matures, and develops its inhibitory and controlling powers, the 'cortical person' arrives. Quoting from the American psychiatrist G. H. Erikson: 'The maturing organism continues after birth to unfold, not new organs but a prescribed sequence of locomotor, sensory and social capacities; which are the material out of which habits and personalities are built. Indeed, this sequence of events appears to be paralleled by a sequence of changes in the electroencephalograms of normal children. In acquiring a social personality the individual is obliged to play many roles. His apprenticeship is served in childhood play, and in adolescence many imaginary roles are discarded and repressed, and the remaining affective roles combined. Not only food and shelter may be matters of life and death – to some individuals it may seem that love and affection are literally vital, and psychologists point out the life-saving function of the mirage principle behind the schizophrenic delusion. By a process of differentiation the subjective ego is built up from the objective unconscious, and this differentiation involves repression and the emergence of consciousness.'

Can we perhaps now formulate the useful question?

How far are conscious processes influenced by homoeopathic potencies? And, as a corollary, are unconscious mental processes to be included in Hahnemann's 'automatic vital force'? Is it reasonable to expect the 'energy' in potencies to produce 'consciousness'?

Let me recall Hahnemann's description of the vital force – or life energy (Paragraph 72), as he also called it. In various paragraphs he describes it as instinctive, irrational, unintelligent, crude, senseless, self-acting, improvident, imperfect, not guided by reason, knowledge or reflection, incapable of any reflection or act of memory, only acting according to the physical constitution. It is clear that Hahnemann excludes conscious activity from the vital force – and yet it is only by guiding what remains of the vital principle in the patient to the proper performance of its functions by means of suitable medicines that cure can be expected. It is true that Hahnemann calls this vital force 'spiritual', but that I believe is because he wishes to emphasise its non-material nature, and he compares its energy with that of gravity and magnetism. The last paragraphs of the *Organon* even refer to the work of Mesmer, Hahnemann's contemporary whose practice laid the foundations for the modern treatment of neuroses. However successful Mesmer was in practice, his theoretical concepts were of no consequence. Mesmer believed that a certain harmony or balance of this 'magnetic fluid' within us always protects us from various ills, and that a disequilibrium causes a variety of illnesses.

Must we consider the 'cortical person' as outside the range of homoeopathic action – functioning at a level that cannot be explained in biochemical or electrophysical terms? Is it possible that only the 'depth person' concerned with essential vital needs – needs that can be expressed in biochemical terms, of oxygen, glucose and the related enzyme systems – is within the sphere of action of homoeopathic potencies? Is our difficulty in treating psychoses therefore bound up with the complications of uncovering and exposing the genetically determined 'depth person', with its stereotyped patterns of behaviour?

Let me recall what Dr Dudgeon wrote in his final lecture: 'In many theoretical points I have dissented from the views of Hahnemann, more especially in regard to his explanation of the curative process, his doctrine of chronic diseases. In these matters Hahnemann may be proved to be in error and yet the truth of the great therapeutical principle with which his name is forever associated is left unaffected.' He continues: 'I am very far from agreeing with those homoeopathic practitioners who see in the doctrines of Hahnemann a perfect and unimprovable system of medicine; on the contrary, I believe there is much, very much to be done.'

We can all join Dudgeon in his exhortation: 'Let us not rest contented with what has been done, but let us each ask ourselves what is still to do and let each contribute his mite towards the great work of reformation so promisingly commenced by Hahnemann.' (*Lectures on the Theory and Practice of Homoeopathy*. Manchester 1854, pp. 559–60).

Chapter 7

Child Psychiatry

My interest in child psychiatry began while I was a houseman at the London Homoeopathic Hospital in 1924, when I spent some of my leisure time attending Dr Crichton-Millar's postgraduate course at the old Tavistock Clinic. Shortly after beginning general practice in Bristol, I was further stimulated by the generous terms of the Leopold Salzburg prize essay and had the honour of the award of the first prize. Subsequent experience convinced me of the importance of neurosis as one of the chief causes of morbidity (not mortality) in general practice. When a few years later it was proposed to start a Child Guidance Clinic in Bristol, I was asked to serve on the committee which organised this service. A few months of membership of this committee convinced me that to be of any service, rather than sit as a figure-head, I should have more practical experience, and so, somewhat to the astonishment of my fellow members, I resigned from the committee and was accepted as a clinical assistant to the new Child Guidance Team. In less than three years World War II had begun, the director of the clinic joined the Army, and I was asked to take over the responsibility of the clinic in his absence.

By the end of the war, the work of the Bristol Clinic had expanded. Two complete teams were working in Bristol and I was also Director of the new Child Guidance Service in Somerset. This was in addition to my duties as senior honorary physician at the Bristol Homoeopathic Hospital.

The experience of working as a member of a team in a child guidance clinic was very stimulating. There was a great deal to learn, and many adjustments to make in the traditional attitude of doctor to patient.

The homoeopathic physician prides himself on his capacity to listen to the patient, down to the minutest detail of all the circumstances of his case, and following Hahnemann, never to cut him short in his description of his sufferings. Nevertheless, in reading the notes prepared by the psychiatric social worker, I realised I was the merest amateur in the art of interviewing, and that to acquire her skill I needed to develop that attitude of acceptance, which neither by word, gesture or expression rejects the patient or what he has to tell.

My empiricism received a cold douche in contact with the scientific precision of the educational psychologist. I learned a little more of the value of evidence, of the risks involved in generalising from clinical experience, and of the importance of proper controls in research. However, continued contact with the psychologists also taught me the limitations of statistical techniques when applied to human problems, and I do not think that the scientific scepticism of the statisticians was ever likely to paralyse the intuitions I had derived from a dozen years of general practice. The emphasis in the early years of child guidance, both in Britain and America, was on the environmental factors responsible for the child's neurotic or delinquent behaviour. It is a surprising fact to realise that the word 'environment' was introduced by Thomas Carlyle in the 19th century. What an all-pervading influence this word has had on our thinking.

In dealing with children, we expect lability of mood and frequent swings from excitement to depression; but when we come to treat the neurotic child, we are confronted with a problem that goes deeper than a temporary change of mood. Recent investigations have emphasised the importance to the infant and young child of continuous loving care from one person. In order to function efficiently, we human beings need a constant internal biochemical state, which may only vary within quite narrow limits – a homoeostasis.

In like manner, if the infant is to develop normally as an individual, he requires an emotional constancy – an emotional homoeostasis during the first two years of life at least. During these early years he develops what has been called 'a central emotional position'. If his first few years have been happy and satisfying, the rest of his life may be devoted to the attempt to recover the emotional climate of that infantile paradise, that Garden of Eden from which we are all excluded once we develop a sense of right and wrong. On the other hand, if the child's original experiences have been unhappy, then he is likely to spend the rest of his life building up defences against this central core of depression.

Even in children this central emotional position is soon buried in the unconscious, and the child is not aware of his emotional state; but various situations and experiences in his subsequent life will trigger off his unconscious search for infantile bliss, or mobilise his defences against infantile depression. Once the unconscious patterns are activated they tend to dominate, so that behaviour becomes rigid and repetitive, and demands become insatiable and unalterable.

If this theory of a central emotional position in the unconscious is valid, it does explain why some stimuli are pathogenic to some children and not to others – why some children can tolerate separation from their mothers without lasting disturbance, while others never recover from the experience. A normal child can digest an extremely traumatic experience in a matter of three months, but the neurotic child's response to external experiences or to internal changes within himself does not necessarily result in a return to equilibrium.

If we are unable to modify or remove the obstacles in his environment that cannot be overcome, what assets can we mobilise? Is it possible to desensitise him to painful stimuli that are unavoidable? Can we make good the discrepancies between the child's ideals and his perhaps inborn inadequacies? I believe we can show that by applying homoeopathic principles it is possible to do just that.

My first example is a boy of nine, referred to me by his family doctor because of sleeplessness and fear of dying. His phobia was not altogether unreasonable, as four years earlier his paternal grandmother – to whom he had been very attached – had died; and now, living in his home, the maternal grandmother was dying of cancer. He was a boy of average intelligence, the oldest of three brothers and very jealous of the next younger brother. Like many children who have had a premature experience of the death of a much-loved relative, he believed that in some way he was responsible for his first grandmother's death, and that somehow his second grandmother's illness was also a punishment for his bad thoughts and deeds. His insomnia was due to his fear of dying himself in his sleep.

I prescribed Phosphorus 30c and he improved, but then he himself fell ill with tonsillitis, and not unnaturally, his previous fears recurred. Spongia helped him and then, as both the boy and grandmother improved, his mother went back to work. This meant that his mother was away from home when he came back from school, and in her absence, he began to be afraid that some accident had befallen her. Once more he relapsed, crying at night, insisting on sleeping with his mother. He improved on Chamomilla, but when his younger brother (and rival) developed whooping cough, and the mother had to have the little boy with her at night time because of the nocturnal paroxysms, he became jealous of this extra attention. Once more, accompanying the jealous feelings, the fear of death recurred.

In view of the series of relapses I decided to give him a deep-acting remedy and ordered a single dose of Sulphur 200c. His mother reported a month later that he was sleeping well in his own room, and no longer made a fuss when she had to leave the house.

This case history illustrates very well the ups and downs of a chronic neurotic, which is what this nine-year-old boy had already become. His grandmother's illness, his own illness, his mother's resumption of work, his brother's illness – each of these events triggered off an acute exacerbation of his chronic neurosis. Although there was a response on each occasion to a homoeopathic remedy, which dealt with the immediate crisis that had been triggered off by the stimulus to which he was oversensitive, it needed a constitutional remedy to establish a satisfactory tolerance to the particular stress – the threat of death and separation – which this neurotic boy found unendurable.

The psychological shock is the factor that releases the crisis, in the same way that the bacterium starts off the infectious illness, or the particular foodstuff determines the allergic reaction; but the underlying cause must be sought in the constitutional weakness of the subject. Even the toughest of us have our breaking point, and if the shocks follow thick and fast, before there is time for a natural recovery, the most robust child is likely to break down.

My next case was a rather delicate boy of nine referred to me by a social worker, again because of the combination of sleeplessness and fear of death. But in this case the family doctor had died and a schoolmate had sustained a fatal road accident, all within four weeks.

His mother had married twice; he had three older half-sibs and was himself the eldest of six children of his mother's second marriage. It is reasonable to point out that all nine children were exposed to the same series of psychological shocks. But this boy was probably the most vulnerable, as he had a history of convulsions, more than one attack of pneumonia, and several attacks of tonsillitis in his first five years.

In this boy's case I ordered a constitutional remedy right away – Sulphur 200c. I think it was a mistake as there was an aggravation, always to be avoided if possible in these neurotic children, but a single dose of Stramonium 200c removed his symptoms. Six months later, the health visitor reported that he was so improved that his mother felt it was unnecessary to bring him to see me again.

My comment on this boy's case is that with these hypersensitive children, staggering under successive shocks, it would be wise to defer the use of a constitutional remedy until the effects of the last trigger situation had been modified by an acute remedy such as Aconite, Belladonna, Chamomilla, Hyoscyamus or Stramonium. An aggravation causing further despair and misery must be avoided at all costs, as it jeopardises any confidence the child or parent may have in the physician.

Grandmothers may die, but sometimes it is as serious a stress if they remain alive. Dorinda, aged ten, was referred to me by her family doctor because of headaches. Her doctor was of the opinion that this was a case of migraine, but a careful investigation of the symptoms as described by the child herself ruled that out. Her mother was anxious, because she herself suffered from migraine and her daughter's headaches were becoming more frequent and severe. The family situation was really dreadful. The child and her mother were tenants of the maternal grandmother, a shocking witchlike creature who delighted in making trouble for her daughter with her malicious gossip, and who swore at her grand-daughter, calling her a liar and accusing her of misdeeds without any foundation. She often threatened to turn mother and child out of the house. Dorinda would not speak to her grandmother and only referred to her as 'she'.

I ordered one dose of Sulphur 30c, and at the end of four weeks only one headache had been reported after an upset at home. I was relieved to learn that shortly afterwards Dorinda's mother left that house and took her away from the baleful influence of the old woman.

Not only can the external environment be responsible for maladjustment, by reason of unpredictable events such as deaths, accidents or rejecting relatives; the internal weather may also be disturbed by volcanic eruptions bursting out without warning from the depths of the self.

Sheila, aged fourteen, was probably the most intelligent girl in Somerset. She had a phenomenal IQ of over 160. She was referred to me by a social worker because of alarming temper outbursts. She was a middle child, envious of her older sister, jealous of her younger brother. Her tantrums were really spectacular, and she frightened her older sister and terrified her mother. Between these outbursts she was a shy, reserved girl with a demure expression. She had won a place at a good school, but after one temper tantrum she was so shockingly rude, not only to her form mistress, but also to her headmistress, that her expulsion was considered. I arranged for an electroencephalogram, and the report came back that this showed a unique abnormality, never previously recorded. Unfortunately, the nature of the abnormal rhythm threw no light on which particular structures were functioning abnormally.

I ordered this clever girl a single dose of Hepar Sulph. 30c. I dared not give a higher potency, as with this remedy the risk of an aggravation had to be avoided at all costs. After this dose the school and family reported that she was a different child – much more willing and helpful in the house, on better terms with her brother, and less likely to 'blow her top' at school. Ten months later there was another outburst at school, but less severe, and one more dose of Hepar Sulph. 30c was prescribed. I had a report from her mother some months later that the improvement had been maintained. I am certain that this intelligent and shy child was swamped from time to time by an emotion of anger so intense that for the time being she was not responsible for her words or deeds. It was only my assurance to her headmistress that I was going to undertake her treatment that saved this promising girl from what would have been a tragic interruption in her school career.

In most neurotic illnesses, even in children, there is no single cause, but a complex interaction between a defective organism and an unfavourable environment. Each step in the development of the neurotic illness leads to a chain reaction of secondary symptoms, which in turn are modified by a feedback mechanism. To sort out this tangle is often bewildering; as one set of symptoms are cleared up, new symptoms take their place, so that a series of remedies appear to be indicated.

Paul, aged ten, was a very obese boy who, when I first saw him, was 58 pounds over the maximum average weight for his age. He was the oldest of three children. His mother had suffered from toxaemia of pregnancy when carrying him; she had great difficulty in weaning him off the bottle, and finally when he was two years old, smashed the feeding bottle deliberately in front of him. A year before I saw him the family had moved from Sussex to a small village in Somerset and he attended the very small local school. Country children are less tolerant of strangers than urban children and this boy was teased unmercifully about his enormous size, and very upset when he was told that he was changing his sex! Indeed, there were some grounds for this rather imaginative threat, as to the uninstructed lay child his minute genitalia were almost concealed by rolls of fat. He was an example of Frölich's syndrome and was referred to me because of enuresis.

I felt that the most important item in the agenda for this boy's programme was to reduce his weight, and accordingly placed him on amphetamine 20mg a day. But in spite of being on one of the orthodox cures for bedwetting at that time, he had a severe relapse of enuresis after six months treatment, and I ordered him a dose of Sulphur 200c. This cleared up the enuresis but reduced his tolerance to the amphetamine drugs, so I had to reduce his dose from 20mg to 5mg a day. However, he continued to lose weight and in a year had lost 12 pounds, and though still looking well-furnished was no longer grossly obese.

Neither was he enuretic, but instead he had resorted to petty pilfering from the larder at home.

A minor deficiency in thyroid production is another type of deficiency resulting in neurotic behaviour.

Peter, aged seven, was a vicar's son, who moved from a quiet country parish to a vicarage situated on a main arterial road in a busy town. All day long he stood at the window, fascinated by the never-ending stream of traffic, and could hardly be persuaded to leave his vantage point to sit down and eat a meal. In school he was dreamy, took no interest in games and made no attempt to make friends. His mother, very deaf, but ambitious for her son, was shocked at his slow progress and consulted the county psychologist, who referred him to me. Without being an obvious cretin, he was sub-thyroid. There was a significant family history. A maternal aunt was a cretin, and a previous child was an encephalic monster. In spite of this sub-thyroidism, confirmed by two consultant paediatricians, he was unable to tolerate an effective dose of thyroid without developing tachycardia, sleeplessness and irritability. After a single dose of Bufo 30c he improved on half the former dose, and at the end of a year a re-test of his intelligence showed a gain of six points (actually an eight per cent gain).

It is often difficult to decide whether the main cause of a neurosis is due to inherited factors, or to exposure to a neurotic parent's demanding and depressing attitudes.

Paul was a sixteen-year-old boy referred to me by the family doctor because he was refusing to attend his grammar school. This was a very serious matter, as that term he was due to take his external examinations. The family doctor had previously referred his father to me. The man was a chronic depressive, a middle-grade civil servant who made everyone's life a misery by his continual moaning and threats of suicide. His wife threatened to leave him, his department threatened to retire him, and his family doctor was utterly fed up with him. It is not difficult to imagine the effect that this unhappy atmosphere had on his unfortunate son, needing as he did to prepare for his examination.

I saw the boy who was himself very insecure and depressed, quite certain of failure, and defeatist about his examination. He defended himself by saying it was all his father's fault; but in many respects he resembled his father, and my impression was that he also was a constitutional depressive. It was impossible to alter the home situation, because although the father toyed with the idea of going into a mental hospital, when it came to the point he jibbed at signing the papers as a voluntary patient.

I could not manipulate the environment, but could I modify the boy's constitution? I prescribed Silica 30c, and a month later his mother reported that he had sat the examination. He was still sure he had failed and I followed up the Silica with a dose of Lycopodium. His father reported six weeks later that he had passed in all subjects, and had decided to leave home. He had been accepted by a bank in another city. His mother confirmed this, saying that the boy was now cheerful and sleeping well.

Now, by contrast, a case illustrating some dangers. Michael, aged eleven, had been referred to me by a surgeon who had admitted him to hospital as a suspected appendix because of repeated vomiting. The surgeon came to the conclusion that the vomiting was functional as it coincided with upsets at school and home. The school reported he was dreamy and his parents said he had fainting attacks.

The only significant history was of a fall off his bicycle. I gave him Arnica 200c, and the following week the parents reported that his head-aches were better but that he was still having attacks of sickness. I then ordered him Natrum Sulph. 30c. Three weeks later the father said the sickness was much better, but that he had had another faint and as he recovered, gabbled a lot of rubbish – fragments of nursery rhymes and so forth. This put me on my guard and I examined his central nervous system and optic discs, without finding anything abnormal. However, I arranged for an electroencephalogram, which was carried out a fortnight later. In that fortnight the boy had developed a left-sided facial weakness and papilloedema of both discs. The electroencephalogram was very abnormal but there were no localising signs in the record. He was placed in the care of a neurosurgeon who operated and found a large astrocytoma of the brain.

To be noted is the temporary effect of the homoeopathic remedies in clearing up the signs of intracranial pressure, the headache and the vomiting. But for the father's chance observation of the confused speech after the faint, which was of course an epileptic phenomenon, I might have let the boy go another month without investigation. As it was, a careful and exhaustive clinical examination revealed nothing at the time, even though the electroencephalogram proved grossly abnormal. We are often accused of treating symptoms, and this last boy is a case in point. But it is interesting to note that in spite of the gross pathology, the homoeopathic potencies had an effect.

As a psychiatrist I have noted an increasing tendency, not only amongst general practitioners but also among consultants, to attribute all kinds of symptoms to psychological causes, after perhaps a very brief history-taking and sometimes after a very cursory physical examination. Time and time again an enuretic child is referred to me and on examination I find undescended testes, indicating delayed development of the urogenital tract, or a coccygeal dimple suggesting a spina bifida occulta. The only psychological aspect is the despair and hopelessness of the young patient, who will have been upbraided and sometimes even punished for his weakness.

Perhaps the most amusing example of this kind of misunderstanding was a boy of eleven, referred to me by a consultant paediatrician for recurrent abdominal pains. He could find no cause for this, decided that they were probably psychological, and sent him to me. I found a rather slow, well-built boy who showed no neurotic features. He was happy at school and appreciated at home, and there were obviously no signs of emotional disturbance. I then interviewed his mother separately, and she confirmed how popular the boy was at school and how well-liked at home. But she said in some ways that he was a funny boy. Naturally I asked for details. 'Well, for one thing', she said, 'he has peculiar tastes. He has a passion for Andrews Liver Salts – he says he likes the flavour and eats it by the spoonful, so I have to hide the tin – in fact, now I lock it up.' Not only homoeopaths have to pay great attention to the smallest details, and be able to recognise the significance of symptoms without getting lost in the minutiae. Treating this boy with Arsenicum Album would not have been the correct management of his problem.

In treating neurotic children we must not only recognise the trigger situations that have precipitated the breakdown, and deal appropriately with them, but we must also detect the fundamental constitutional weaknesses, whether inherited or built in by the experiences of the first few months of life. We must not only desensitize the individual to the bombardment of stimuli that cannot be avoided (the bombers always get through), but mobilise such assets in the constitution as will help to bridge the gap between the patient's inadequacies and his ideals.

Chapter 8

Psychiatric Disorders of Old Age

The medical problems of elderly people are often left untreated. Such patients will tell me that their family practitioner has said, 'Look Gran, it's your age, you must learn to live with it.'

It is this therapeutic hopelessness that the homoeopath must be prepared to combat. We need the optimism of a Burnett. Dr Burnett had been brilliantly successful in curing a case of panophthalmitis in less than twenty-four hours, and his grateful patient then asked him, 'If this is what homoeopathy can do, could you cure my cataract?' Dr Burnett was no specialist in eye diseases, and from the nature of the complaint he thought he could hardly expect to influence it. Two London specialists had diagnosed the cataract but had stated that it was not ripe enough for operation. Burnett however agreed with the patient's request to try and cure her cataract with homoeopathic medicines. He saw the patient once a month and at the end of a year, after a variety of homoeopathic prescriptions, the opacities in her lens had disappeared and she had recovered her vision.

Senile cataract is an example of an old age process, and it is therefore instructive to note the remedies that Burnett subsequently used in treating other cases (I exclude the congenital, diabetic and traumatic cataracts from his case histories). The best results followed the use of such constitutional remedies as Sulphur, Silica, Phosphorus, Calc. Carb.; other remedies found useful were Causticum, Conium and Lycopodium. As Burnett emphasizes, cataract is a constitutional complaint; it is essential to treat the patient, not the cataract.

I highlight this old age process of cataract as an example of the many problems of senility. We should recognise at once that the majority of our elderly patients have often three or more different lesions at the same time.

Examples are a lady of 81 with a blood pressure of 240/85, angina of effort, osteoarthritis of the spine, diurnal frequency of micturition; or a gentleman of 75 with prolapse of the rectum, diverticulitis and hiatus hernia. A lady of 70, with coronary thrombosis, congestive heart failure, cataracts in both eyes and bilateral osteoarthritis of the hips. A gentleman of 85 with an adenoma of the thyroid, auricular fibrillation, a corkscrew oesophagus and an inguinal hernia. I will briefly describe the last case as an illustration of the prescribing problems.

The large adenoma of the thyroid disappeared in a few months after a course of repeated doses of Spongia. The dysphagia due to the abnormal oesophagus reacted quite quickly to Arsenicum Album given just before meals; but then this patient was hit by a small pulmonary embolism. He looked very ill indeed, but Bryonia 200c cleared up the pain and fever in less than 24 hours. After this episode he showed signs of congestive heart failure, with oedema of the legs, scrotum and prepuce. Apis gave relief, but I noted that in spite of being successful, none of these prescriptions had any influence on the auricular fibrillation, which required material doses of digitalis to control. Nevertheless, with homoeopathic treatment, all of these handicapped patients are mobile, move about the country and follow their interests and hobbies.

We need to ask what is normal to expect of our elderly patients. While many surveys have been reported from geriatric and mental hospitals, I find the pioneer work of Sheldon in Wolverhampton particularly useful, as he organised his enquiries on subjects living in their own homes or with relatives.

Of the women of 85 or over, he found more than two-thirds had a defect of hearing, nearly 7 out of 10 were liable to tumble, 7 out of 10 suffered from vertigo, and 9 out of 10 had difficulty in getting about in the dark. The failure in recalling surnames he regarded as normal.

Sheldon classified the old people according to their mental state. Class I he assessed as fully normal mentally and these comprised 82 per cent of the total number. Class II had faculties slightly impaired; they were subject to mood changes, easy tears, easy laughter, temper tantrums; inclined to be resentful and suspicious. He considered most of them had previously been of dull intelligence, some of them even subnormal; these accounted for 11 per cent of his group. We would think first of Barium salts for the intellectually dull. Baryta Carb. has fear, particularly of strangers, and is suspicious. Nux Moschata has tears alternating with laughter as an outstanding symptom.

Sheldon's Class III included the forgetful, the childish who were difficult to live with; there were only 3 per cent of these. Again Baryta Carb. has both childishness and forgetfulness, but other remedies to be borne in mind are Cicuta and Carboneum Sulph. Cicuta is notable for its twitchings, jerks and convulsions, and its tendency to skin eruptions.

Carbon. Sulph. has the flatulence of Carbo Veg. and the abdominal soreness of Sulphur; disturbances of vision are quite a feature; defective memory and inability to find the right word are also among its symptoms.

The last of Sheldon's classes, Class IV, are the demented, but this was a very small class of not quite 1 per cent. The severe deterioration was manifested by the gross forgetfulness, the slow speech, the restlessness and agitation, the contrariness, the malicious resentment, the suspicion, the dislike of being left alone, the tendency to hoard. Remedies to consider for these cases are Argentum Nit., Mercurius and Tarentula. The Argentum Nit. patients are worse at night; they look withered and dried up. Mercurius too is worse at night, but is sensitive to changes of both hot and cold; sweats and salivation and dribbling are a marked feature, and so is tremor. Characteristic of Tarentula are the congested facies, the dysphagia, the choreic movements and the extreme restlessness. This restlessness is aggravated by a barbiturate or other sedative, which diminishes what cortical control remains in these demented patients. There is a parallel with the hyperkinetic children whose behaviour is aggravated by barbiturates and improved by amphetamines – which stimulate the cerebral cortex, as child psychiatrists have discovered.

Sheldon pointed out that deterioration in these old people into a lower class of function may follow a fall, and quotes two cases that became more demented, one following a fall downstairs, and another after being knocked down by a car.

The pathological changes in the brain of these senile patients are attributed to the development of senile plaques in the cerebral cortex. This involves the loss of irreplaceable cells, but Roth points out that senile plaques are to be found in normal old people; in senile dementia they are much more numerous. Electron microscope studies suggest that senile plaques involve the destruction of dendrites, synapses and axons, with the formation of abnormal proteins of an amyloid nature. Other biochemical changes may also be implicated.

Not only are these senile patients handicapped by a defective cortex, but in addition a Canadian psychiatrist has shown that their adrenal cortex over-reacts to provocation. Experience at the Crichton Royal Hospital has shown that elderly organic patients are extremely sensitive to drugs; many of them quickly develop signs of toxicity which, though not dramatic, may have an insidious fatal outcome. This alone is a powerful argument for attempting relief with homoeopathic remedies. Forrsmann of Sweden has warned against the risks of going too fast with modern drug therapy in these older patients. He reminds us of the possibilities of epileptic seizures and the frequent development of extrapyramidal symptoms of parkinsonism when using phenothiazines; of the vascular symptoms of raised blood pressure after monoamine oxidase inhibitors when used as antidepressants. Attention has also been drawn to the sudden deaths in patients taking tricyclic antidepressants.

Depression in old age raises another important topic. The depressives are the exception to the rule that patients with chronic brain disease show brain changes such as senile plaques. Depressive illness is the commonest psychiatric illness in old age. One survey showed that 12 per cent of patients over 65 suffered from a psychiatric illness; and 60 per cent of these had a depressive illness, compared with 40 per cent who had a degenerative disease of the brain.

It is important to recognise these depressives, because the great majority of them are curable. Roth gives a dramatic illustration. When he first worked in a mental hospital twenty-five years before, he recalled an old lady of 79 who drew attention to her presence in a chronic ward by setting fire to her hair; she had been in the hospital for ten years, having initially been diagnosed as suffering from senile dementia. She proved to be suffering from a severe endogenous depression; she made an excellent response to electroconvulsive therapy (ECT) and was discharged to live with her daughter.

My present case-load includes fifty-eight patients of pensionable age. Of these, no less than twelve have suffered from depressive illnesses; some of them have previously been on antidepressant drugs or subjected to ECT. Two of them were so severely depressed that they could not be managed at home and had to be transferred to mental hospitals. These depressives do not always present as psychiatric patients. One octogenarian consulted me originally about her cataract; a 67-year-old man asked for help about his osteoarthritis; another man in his late sixties complained of hay fever; a 70-year-old man approached me about his senile pruritus; a 60-year-old lady was harrassed by a laryngeal tic, another 69-year-old lady grumbled about vague abdominal pains, another of the same age about backache; a 70-year-old man about recurrent bronchitis, and a 64-year-old woman about hyperpiesia. Only three of the dozen admitted depression as the presenting symptom, although a detailed history demonstrated previous depressive phases in seven of these patients.

As you would expect in such an assortment, no one remedy was indicated for these depressives, but I found Platina, Argentum Nit., Nux Vomica, Psorinum, Lycopodium and Natrum Mur. were useful when indicated by the symptoms. While the majority of my patients were suffering from recurrent depressions of the endogenous type, there was a smaller group of reactive depressions. One woman in her late sixties had suffered a cardiac arrest under an anaesthetic, and her abdomen had to be closed with gallstones still in situ. How far the anoxia consequent on the cardiac arrest was responsible, how far the shock of her very close call, which her husband had not been able to conceal from her, had contributed to her mental reaction, it is difficult to estimate; but from a lively and popular hostess of a big country house, she had given up her busy social life and sat silent by the fireside.

Another woman was a tall asthenic subject who had recently lost her husband from a coronary thrombosis; she responded to Ignatia and Natrum Mur. and made good progress for two years, but relapsed after her greenhouse was wrecked by vandals; bereft of her occupational therapy, she needed Ignatia and Natrum Mur. again and made a good recovery.

But the recent loss of a spouse is not the only cause of social desolation and social isolation; the departure of children to marry and live in a different part of the country or even abroad, or to be the sole survivor of one's siblings, can equally contribute to loneliness and chronic grief.

For these reactive depressions caused by bereavement, we think of Aurum, Causticum or Cocculus, especially when the bereavement has been preceded by a protracted period of nursing. Ignatia when the depressive broods in silence, Lachesis and Natrum Mur. for the patients who cannot cry. Phosphoric Acid and Staphysagria, particularly the latter, when the bereaved partner feels an irrational resentment at the departure, indeed the desertion by death of his or her partner.

Orthodox practitioners have noted that on prescribing tricyclic antidepressants there may be a time-lag of as much as three weeks before the drug appears to act. I have found a rapid response after Ignatia, but I have noted that improvement after Aurum and Natrum Mur. may not be noticed for ten or more days; it is characteristic of Natrum Mur. that these patients are reluctant to admit improvement.

It requires some judgement to decide, on the severity of the depression, whether to switch to an antidepressant drug; but I have no hesitation in recommending inpatient treatment for the actively suicidal. To leave such a patient at home is an unfair responsibility to place on the family.

So far we have considered senility with cerebral predominance, and we have also identified the depressive illnesses of the aged. But we still have to consider the toxic delirious reactions of old age. These acute confusions are often associated with vascular pathology; less frequently with an acute infection, metabolic disturbances, drug intoxication, hypothermia or uraemia. Metabolic disturbances include hypoglycaemia when glucose metabolism is upset in old age.

Myxoedema sometimes can give rise to a confused state; it is important to recognise mild degrees of hypothyroidism, as it is readily treatable. Recent research on immunity also suggests that thyroid reinforces some of the natural defence mechanisms, and the inference could be that thyroid could be prescribed at the same time as the homoeopathic remedy.

It is important to discover what drugs the confused patient has previously been taking, or even though the identification of the assortment of tablets and capsules produced by anxious relatives can be a problem.

Hypothermia may be aggravated by the previous prescription of sedatives. It is easy to kill such a patient by warming her up too rapidly. I would suggest that on the symptomatology of cold abdomen, cold thighs, gruff voice, stiff neck, slurred speech and coarse tremor, Camphor is a remedy to be considered.

The more common cause of delirium in the aged is arterial disease leading to ischaemic destruction of the brain cells, i.e. arteriosclerotic dementia.

Delirium is the most frequent symptom, often occurring at night, when it is most disturbing in the hospital ward. Mayer-Gross has shown that this delirium can be reproduced when these senile patients are placed in a dark room. It is interesting to note that Kent's *Repertory* lists Calc. Ars., Carbo Veg., Cuprum and Stramonium under 'Delirium in the dark'.

Nocturnal delirium and restlessness is often associated with diurnal drowsiness, and on a ward round the next morning it is difficult to believe that the somnolent patient had been noisy and overactive, hallucinated and disorientated in time and place. These arteriosclerotic psychoses often have a sudden onset compared with the slow deterioration seen in the Alzheimer type of primary neurone destruction.

Loss of orientation in the dark must be a frightening experience for these patients, giving rise to a feeling of helplessness; this impotent fear is often joined by or gives rise to anger, and the angry person then fears retaliation, so that paranoid elements in his thinking soon develop and he is suspicious of all attempts to help him. Bearing in mind that delirious patients are often hallucinated, drowsy by day, or doubly incontinent, I think first of Hyoscyamus, as well as Belladonna, Arsenicum, Lachesis, Secale, Veratrum and Stramonium.

I have found Belladonna of most value in robust overweight indivi-

51

duals. In the delirious state Belladonna has a fear of imaginary animals. Stramonium, which also has a flushed face, is more afraid of being hurt and panics at the sight of the hypodermic syringe, whereas Hyoscyamus is usually pale; the Hyoscyamus patient tends to tear up her clothes and take them off, and there is a sexual element in this behaviour. Arsenicum is too chilly to unclothe, but Lachesis will undo clothing or throw it off because she cannot tolerate any constriction around her body; Lachesis is nearly always cyanosed, and refuses medicine because she is afraid of being poisoned. Lachesis wakes out of sleep into a delirious state, complains that the ward is so stifling hot that she will get out of bed to try and force the windows open.

The Secale patient wants cold because of the burning pains in the extremities; Secale is generally a decrepit, wrinkled subject with pulseless arteries in the legs and feet and a tendency to gangrene of the toes.

Finally a few comments on the cerebral sequelae of a stroke. Dr Tyler recorded a dramatic result in a patient comatose after a stroke. A woman of 80 with cerebral thrombosis, paralysed and comatose for nine weeks; the coma had become so deep that it was almost impossible to get a mouthful of anything down. The consultant advised Nux Moschata; a single dose of the 200th potency was prescribed and the patient promptly recovered consciousness, living on for another five years in full possession of her faculties.

In hemiplegic patients we often see residual disabilities of considerable gravity: the loss of very recent memory must be borne in mind. Such patients forget the instructions of the nurse, the physiotherapist and the speech therapist, and the risk is that they will be labelled uncooperative.

Then there are the patients who exhibit a cheerful air of unconcern after a stroke, which should make us think of Opium or Arnica; or they will deny ownership of the paralysed limb, a symptom sometimes observed when the right temporal lobe has been involved. This is not the feverish symptom of the Baptisia patient, who has the sensation of limbs scattered over the bed, but it will be found in the symptom lists of Silica, Petroleum and Agaricus, all of which have this disturbance of the body-image. Indeed, Agaricus is so unaware of her disability that she will try to get out of bed; these are patients who should be nursed in a cot. Intensive physiotherapy is necessary to combat their neglect of the paralysed anaesthetic limb and to restore some function to the apraxic hand. The postural instability and frequent falls result in a loss of confidence, and patients give up too easily.

Kent writes that once the coma following a cerebral haemorrhage has been relieved by Opium he relies on Plumbum, Phosphorus and Alumina. The Plumbum patient typically has a dry yellowish wrinkled skin, has a partial aphasia, is constipated; tends to exaggerate her disabilities until her relatives suspect her of malingering. The Phosphorus patient has much more drive to recover; typically a pale face with blue rings round the eyes; is thirsty, better for eating; likes to be rubbed, enjoys her physiotherapy sessions; the ophthalmoscope reveals retinal haemorrhages. The Alumina patient is like the Plumbum patient in that he is constipated; has difficulty in passing even a soft stool; prefers dry food in spite of dry mucous membranes; there can be depersonalisation and derealisation; familiar surroundings seem strange.

Finally, a reminder that we must take the total situation into account. I remember a 70-year-old retired headmistress who lived alone in the country. She had made a recovery from a cerebral thrombosis and a depressive illness; she complained of severe pains in her legs, and with some reluctance she unrolled her stockings to display the petechiae and subcutaneous haemorrhages of scurvy. I did not hesitate to prescribe large doses of ascorbic acid.

Dr Irene Rogers has emphasized the importance of adequate feeding. 'If more doctors would visit their patients instead of handing out pills, and would go and look in the kitchen, they would see the answer to some of their questions. Some of their patients will have ghastly old stoves on which they cannot cook; while in modern old peoples' homes there may be a super modern electric stove which they cannot work; they can switch it on but they cannot see whether it is hot or cold.'

Someone said that there are three ways of growing old – resigning, denying, or accepting. As homoeopathic physicians, it should be our function to make it easier for our elderly patients to accept their limitations and to prescribe for them so as to reduce those limitations to the minimum.

Chapter 9

Hypertension in the Elderly

Many patients over fifty in a general practice will be found to be exhibiting a raised blood pressure. For present purposes I define the lower limits as 160mm systolic and 90mm diastolic. What kind of people develop hypertension? There is some argument about the importance of heredity, but Platt considers it a specific inherited disorder of middle age. He points out that the parents and siblings of patients with essential hypertension suffer in the same way, and that their younger brothers and sisters, as they reach middle age, show a rise in blood pressure.

Specialists in psychosomatic medicine have summarised the characteristics of the personality developing essential hypertension. Compared with other types of patient, they have an extremely high record of previous illness. In temperament they are predominantly introverts. Many of them have neurotic symptoms and bottle up their feelings, which if they do find expression, do so in an explosion. They are ambitious but fear they will fail, and so select an occupation below their real capacity. There is a continual conflict between active and passive roles. They would like to identify with authority figures, but on the other hand need to be taken care of. Because of this ambivalence, they have difficulty in making decisions. When they discover or learn that they have high blood pressure, their feelings are a mixture of fear, exaggerated fear of a stroke or paralysis, and relief that they have an excuse for failing to attain their ambitions or goals. To tell these patients not to worry is absurd. Even if you ask them if they are worried about anything, they will say 'No', because often they do not realise how deeply disturbed they are; but they will, once they know about their blood pressure, project their worries on to that.

To consider the psychosomatic profile, here are a collection of mental symptoms. If one attempts to look them up in Kent's *Repertory*, some equivalents must be accepted:

Timidity (shyness)

Oversensitive (sensitive to criticism)

Lack of self-confidence
Irresolution (cannot make decisions)
Effects of grief

When these are repertorised, the remedy which is best represented is Lycopodium, and other remedies which come through are Aurum, Ignatia, Sulphur and Natrum Muriaticum. But these are mental symptoms only, and in finding the simillimum one has to take into consideration other symptoms and other modalities. There is evidence of hereditary factors – the well-defined pattern of psychological attitudes indicate that in essential hypertension we are dealing with a particular type of constitution, and we are therefore encouraged to rely on constitutional remedies in treating this condition.

The history of the homoeopathic treatment of essential hypertension belongs to the twentieth century: sphygmomanometers were not routinely used in general practice much before the 1920s. The first reference I can find to essential hypertension in homoeopathic literature is a note by an American physician in 1924 who, however, had no suggestions about suitable remedies. It was not until 1931 that two French homoeopaths recommended Baryta Carb. and Plumbum, not forgetting Ignatia for the temporary hypertension which they noted tended to follow emotional shocks.

From the sixties onwards, in contrast to the 1930s, the problem has become more complicated. The majority of patients will already have had orthodox treatment for hypertension; and often it is because the side effects proved so troublesome that they have asked for a further opinion. For example, one man was referred to me, as a psychiatrist, because of his depression. It emerged that he had been prescribed reserpine for hypertension, and that he had developed the characteristic depression – one of the side effects of Rauwolfia, from which reserpine is derived. Depression was observed in the provings of Rauwolfia by the London Faculty of Homoeopathy. It was difficult to persuade him to discontinue his reserpine as he had been so alarmed by the discovery of a raised blood pressure. Actually his raised blood pressure was desirable, because he suffered from polycythaemia and his heart required more force to pump the viscous blood through his arteries. His blood pressure was contained within normal limits with spaced doses of Cobalt 30c, which was prescribed not so much for the hypertension as for his raised blood count.

A more troublesome group of toxic reactions follows the use of methyldopa. Some 20–25% of patients cannot tolerate this drug – 20%

of them develop a positive Coombs test in three to six months, and this reaction takes six months to disappear after discontinuing the drug. This positive test is the preliminary stage of a subsequent haemolytic anaemia; but not only are the red cells attacked – cases of agranulocytosis have also been reported. Further, the action of methyldopa is potentiated by very powerful diuretics such as hydrochlorothiazide, so much so that some authorities have considered there is a risk of cerebral and cardiac ischaemia using this combination.

A septuagenarian lady came to see me. She lived alone in a large country house which she had divided up into flats; her married son lived in another part of the house. Petite and wrinkled, she stumbled across my consulting room, complaining of giddiness, faintness, headaches and lack of concentration. She had a blood pressure of 230/115, and she showed me her collection of at least four different drugs. For the immediate severe vertigo I ordered her Cocculus, and after she had time to accustom herself to the absence of the powerful drugs, I gave her spaced doses of Sulphur 30c, then 200c. Her blood pressure hardly varied in the six months afte discontinuing the chlorothiazides, but she felt so much better in herself that she was able to resume her gardening and to go out by herself, which she had been afraid to do before. I heard no more from her for six months until she asked me to prescribe for an attack of shingles.

Why Sulphur in this particular case? She certainly was not the Sulphur stereotype of the 'ragged philosopher'. Her outstanding symptoms, once she was clear of side effects, were faintness on standing, and burning in the feet, which was so intense that she could not keep them still, trying to find a cool place in the sheets. Sulphur has these two symptoms strongly, and further enquiry elicited other symptoms characteristic of Sulphur. It is worth noting that at the end of six months, when she was obviously so much better, her blood pressure was still over 200. Just concentrating on lowering her blood pressure was not going to help this lady. Indeed it has been pointed out that despite pharmacological control of blood pressure, patients still get strokes. Atherosclerosis and damaged endothelium are therefore also of importance, even if the blood pressure is within the normal range.

I cite as an example an octogenarian, a huge man of over six feet, weighing 18 stone. In his time he had been a very high-powered executive indeed, on Christian name terms with cabinet ministers and ambassadors. He developed giant-celled arteritis, which is not necessarily associated with raised blood pressure. A second opinion was sought, and because of the risk of blindness, steroids were recommended. After six months these were tailed off, but this patient developed sudden losses of memory lasting several hours. In these amnesias he enquired after his wife who had been dead for some years, and did not recognise his surroundings, demanding to be taken to the country house which he had given up a decade ago. Belladonna 200c proved to be the most effective remedy for this condition, clearing up the amnesia in an hour. But while this short-acting remedy proved efficient, it was much more difficult to treat his general condition, even six months after the steroids had been entirely discontinued. Apparently well-indicated remedies such as Calcarea Carb. and Baryta Carb. did not relieve his general discontented attitude, the slight stiffness of hemiplegic distribution, or the slight apraxia. It is hard to estimate how far the course of steroids had upset his autoimmune reactions.

Some of the most difficult problems are presented by the patient who cannot accept a diagnosis and runs from one doctor to another. I think of one married woman whom I first saw seven years ago, who consulted me for migraine and for what she had been informed was cholecystitis. Before consulting me she had had treatment from an osteopath, a naturopath, an unqualified psychologist and an eye specialist. She was a stout woman, very accident-prone, very sorry for herself, who wrote every month a long-winded diary of her fluctuating symptoms. Her migraine symptoms appeared to indicate Phosphorus, but after a month's treatment with little improvement, she wrote saying that she was accustomed to take a whole range of proprietary salts, and would any of these clash with my treatment? She was shocked when I recommended that she discontinued the lot.

In view of such an accumulation of medicines, I next ordered her a dose of Sulphur 30c to attempt to clear the picture. Her next report showed little improvement and I found that in the meanwhile, impatient with her slow progress, she had bought herself some tonic and fallen back on previous supplies of laxatives and ergotamine preparations. She was very hurt when I remonstrated with her, and a month later took umbrage when I had unavoidably to postpone a consultation. The picture was still a very confused one, and I repeated the Sulphur, this time 200c. She began to miss appointments and I suggested that, as she appeared to have lost confidence, perhaps she would do better to seek other advice. I heard no more from her for some years until she appeared once more asking for an appointment, as now she had been to see a consultant in her home town who told her she had raised blood pressure. When I had originally seen her her systolic had been under 150, but now it was 170. Her consultant had given her a regime of methyldopa, valium and antihistamine. On this combination she felt worse and had come back to me for advice. Once more I warned her that homoeopathic treatment would be a waste of time for her unless she was prepared to discard the allopathic treatments; once more I ordered Sulphur, and was prepared for the rise in blood pressure to 210 when she came to see me again. But in herself she was feeling better. I do not consider that Sulphur is this patient's constitutional remedy. I prescribed it on the advice that it will clear a confused picture.

What is notable about this patient is her impatience and impulsiveness. In the seven years I have known her she has moved house four times and changed her family doctor as often. Remedies characterised by impatience are Chamomilla, Ignatia, Nux Vomica, Sepia and Sulphur. Impulsive remedies are Argentum Nit., Arsenicum Alb., Aurum and Cicuta. Perhaps Aurum will prove to be her remedy.

Aurum was the remedy for another woman, also heavily built. She had been a missionary in the Far East, but was expelled and returned to the United Kingdom. She was a woman of enormous energy who wrote books, edited a magazine and worked part-time as a librarian. As is so often typical of the hypomaniac, she wrote immensely lengthy letters, running to five sheets of foolscap. She was liable to depressed phases, when her blood pressure tended to rise near the 200 mark. I prescribed Aurum on the combination of suicidal thoughts, her fidgety restlessness, hot flushes and her state of being in a hurry. She responded well to a few spaced doses and her blood pressure fell some 40 points.

When the raised blood pressure is an accompaniment of a serious heart condition, such as the past history of a coronary thrombosis, it is again important to take the whole person into consideration rather than to concentrate on the blood pressure alone.

The managing director of a family business, who had recently been discharged from hospital after a coronary thrombosis, came to see me. He had been given a guarded prognosis by his cardiologist and was very depressed, convinced that he had only a year to live; he was neurotic, sleeping badly, and conscious of his heart beat. He had been prescribed propranolol and a potassium supplement. When I saw him his blood pressure was 200/120. He was a pale sallow man, easily exhausted, short of breath, very sensitive to cold air; he found it difficult to concentrate on his office work, and was troubled with flatulent distension which persisted after burping. I gave him China and in six months his pressure had dropped to 150/95 and he had been able to resume his hobbies. Naturally in his case I checked his pulse pressure and systolic/diastolic ratio carefully, as it is important to maintain an adequate circulation through the coronary arteries.

Anxiety over the possibility of another coronary thrombosis may be a factor in raising the blood pressure; another cause for anxiety is the fear of blindness. When this is combined with a tendency to recurrent depressions, the problem becomes formidable. I have known one such patient for forty years, who in that time has been in hospital some half-dozen times because of depressive phases. Concerned even when well about her failing sight, due to cataracts, she nevertheless was immensely independent, and after her husband's death lived by herself until well over eighty, refusing help from her devoted son and daughter-in-law, and critical of the social worker who did her best to persuade her to take up residence in a home for the partially-sighted. Having known her and her husband for many years, I continued to treat her on a friendly basis, but she would never accept this arrangement and insisted on paying me a token fee. This very proud old woman was a typical Platinum. She felt herself superior to her neighbours, whom she despised. As an old woman she became shaky, but disregarded her trembling hands; she was dark, thin, stiff, disliked company. From time to time she would disappear into a mental hospital or geriatric ward, but would discharge herself and ask me to visit her, when she grumbled quite unjustifiably about the treatment she had experienced. Platinum usually gave her some relief.

This last case was an endogenous depression, but the reactive depressions also tend to develop raised blood pressures.

I had under care a middle-aged woman who had lost her husband two years previously; she was left responsible for an older bachelor brother-in-law who had shared the house. The brother-in-law became more and more of an invalid. He finally developed diabetic gangrene and was admitted to hospital for amputation. When the hospital social worker informed my patient that the surgeon was discharging her octogenarian brother-in-law back to her house, she could not sleep or eat, lost two stone in weight in a very short time, and developed severe headaches. I found she had a blood pressure of over 200 systolic. She was a thin, willowy woman with a scraggy neck, still mourning for her husband, disliking company and sympathy. After a single dose of Natrum Mur. 1M her blood pressure dropped to 160 systolic, but rose again when her brother-in-law had to undergo a second amputation at a distant hospital and she felt it her duty to make the effort to journey to visit him. Ignatia was prescribed with effect.

In contrast, a sexagenarian lady was a much tougher proposition. For some two years she nursed her mother, who was dying slowly from an oesophageal stricture. Soon after her mother's death, her husband developed a hemiplegia and her role as a nurse continued; but added to this she took over the management of her husband's business as a building contractor, and continued to do this after his death. Twenty years earlier her blood pressure was 150, but after her husband's stroke it rose to 185. At this time she was obviously overworked and under great pressure; she forgot what she had to do, her sleep was often interrupted and unrefreshing and she woke with severe headaches. In my consulting room she moved her chair away from the fire and asked for the window to be opened. She was accustomed to keep herself going with lots of spirits. Such physical symptoms as she had were left-sided. Lachesis 30c was of considerable assistance, and a year later her systolic pressure had dropped to 140.

The last case is one of hypertensive encephalopathy. This was a huge old man who in his time rode in point-to-points and had only recently given up his stables and riding to hounds. Ten years ago I had found his blood pressure 220/125 and had prescribed Sulphur 200c for him. He made a second marriage at seventy-five and moved out of the district; but recently I was asked to see him again. He was now bedridden and liable to fits, preceded by bouts of hiccoughs and followed by prolonged bouts of coughing. His blood pressure had hardly varied from ten years previously. Although he was a sociable man, striking symptoms were that he was worse for conversation and got very flushed when talking. He had a sensation of falling through the bed; his skin tended to an oily perspiration, and he had an aversion to hot drinks. I ordered him China 30c and told his wife that when his leg began to jerk, which was the prodromal sign of a fit, to give him Stramonium 30c every quarter-hour. In the next four months he had only two slight fits, which were quickly over, and until his wife was involved in a serious car accident was very much better.

The point to be made is that in dealing with essential hypertension, the long-acting results depend on identifying the constitutional remedy of the patient as a whole, rather than finding a remedy for the blood pressure by itself.

Chapter 10

Rheumatic Diseases

Patients who complain of 'rheumatism' are a very mixed bunch. Some of them have diagnosed themselves, others have had unsuccessful treatment elsewhere, and quite a number have had private treatment from physiotherapists. As homoeopathic physicians, we tend to be the last resort when everything and everybody has failed. Perhaps this is the reason why we see more unusual cases than most doctors – some of these patients are suffering from rare and uncommon syndromes.

In a typical twelve months of practice, I saw twenty-five rheumatic patients; besides osteoarthritis, rheumatoid arthritis, menopausal arthritis and cervical spondylosis, I have had cases of lumbago, sciatica, frozen shoulder, gout, bursitis, giant-celled arteritis, post-gastrectomy osteomalacia, polymyalgia rheumatica, chronic abortus infection, gross obesity (over 21 stone), and two cases of long-distance motorists with badly adjusted driving seats and control pedals.

Thirteen different remedies were used: Actaea, Bryonia, Calcarea Carb., Colocynth, Lachesis, Lycopodium, Natrum Mur., Psorinum, Ruta, Sepia, Silica and Sulphur. The three remedies I found indicated most frequently, and which were followed by the best results, are: Bryonia, Calcarea Carb. and Rhus Tox.

My Bryonia cases were generally examples of osteoarthritis of the hips; they were all over sixty; they had marked radiological evidence of bony changes in the heads of the femora and acetabula with well-developed osteophytes. Two of them needed two sticks to walk with, and one used elbow crutches. Because of coincident cardiac pathology the surgeons had refused operations on two patients for replacement of hip joints. The prognosis for relief of pain did not appear very promising, yet Bryonia gave very considerable relief – so much so that one old lady could discard both her sticks and one elderly gentleman gave up his elbow crutch.

One does not expect to make any changes in the radiological appearances of the bony structures around the joints. It must be

61

supposed that the main action of Bryonia is on muscles in protective spasm, guarding over-protectively against movement in the disintegrated joint, and giving rise to more pain and spasm on any movement.

Bryonia is one of the remedies of antiquity and was recommended by Dioscorides. Hahnemann proved it with six assistants; he pointed out its similarity in action to Rhus Tox., but showed that it was the opposite to Rhus as far as the modality of motion was concerned. Bryonia is always worse from any motion and better for rest – whereas Rhus is always worse for rest and better after the first movement. Hahnemann commented on the alternating action of Bryonia, recommending that if there is no response in the first twenty-four hours the dose – and he used very high potencies – should be repeated.

Hughes emphasised the action of Bryonia on serous membranes and used it in rheumatic fever. Royal said the sour sweat of rheumatic fever was a typical Bryonia symptom; he also used it in osteoarthritis. Clarke quotes Teste that Bryonia is suitable for persons who overeat, who eat excessively of meat and are accustomed to rich living. He emphasises the need of the Bryonia patient to keep still; of Bryonia's relation to other remedies; Clarke says it is close to Calcarea Carb., so that they must never be prescribed one after the other. Clarke says the chronic of Bryonia is Alumina; certainly, both remedies share constipation with large dry hard stool.

Kent says that in contrast to Aconite, Bryonia illnesses develop slowly; he considers Bryonia patients are upset by eating vegetable salads and sauerkraut; he advises that you should not cross a Bryonia patient – it will make him worse. Neatby and Stonham emphasise the aggravation from movement, the relief from rest; pressure aggravates, so that there is pain in the heel or sole when walking, from the weight of the body; they point out that the Bryonia patient is irritable and cannot take any opposition, is easily upset by controversy or disappointment; typically has dark hair and complexion and the muscles are firm and fleshy.

As an example, I had under my care a very rich man of eighty who had a post-gastrectomy osteomalacia, and who was so crippled that he depended on an elbow crutch. He was much worse from movement, was easily upset and extremely irritable. He decided that he was suffering from arthritis, and found it hard to accept that an orthopaedic surgeon refused to consider him for operation. He insisted on having a third opinion, and a series of investigations demonstrated his loss of calcium; in the meanwhile he had considerable relief from Bryonia.

In my series, Rhus Tox. proved to be the next most frequently indicated remedy and the next most successful. Rhus was introduced in 1798 by a French doctor as a treatment for herpes. Hahnemann pointed out that the pains of Bryonia and Rhus are similar, but that they could be distinguished easily because the Rhus patient has the severest symptoms and sufferings when at rest. Severe rigidity and pain is experienced on first moving the joints after rest, as on waking in the morning, but after the joints are moved for a while the pain is lessened.

Hughes considers that the stiffness is more of a handicap than the pain; the patients constantly shift their position. Clarke points out the restlessness of Rhus; the pain and soreness are better by movement. Royal confirms the stiffness. After many years of experience, Hahnemann considered it was the most efficacious remedy for the effects of overlifting or the inordinate exertion of muscles.

Clarke says a common cause is stretching up high to reach things. Wheeler says the pains will return if movement is continued until fatigue comes on; he claims that the pains are worse at night because of the enforced rest in bed. Neatby and Stonham state that the pain in bed may be so bad that the Rhus patient has to get out and walk about the bedroom. Clarke is of the opinion that damp is a provoking factor, especially damp sheets. Wheeler says damp is more deleterious to the Rhus patient than cold winds, to which Rhododendron patients are very susceptible. Kent speaks of the aggravation from cold damp air, and that taking a bath will stop the action of Rhus. Gibson Miller claims that camphor antidotes Rhus, so patients should be discouraged from rubbing the affected parts with camphorated oil or analgesic creams containing camphor. Hahnemann warns that amelioration of symptoms is not to be expected for twenty-four hours; he advises that Rhus should not be prescribed in a lower potency than the 30th.

Wheeler states that Radium has a similar symptomatology to Rhus but a deeper action. If a patient has responded to Rhus a little, but remains uncured, Radium will often complete the cure, as in the following case.

A sixty-year-old widow, with brown hair not yet grey, and blue eyes, complained that she could not put her right arm behind her back, that her left knee tended to give out; that the pain at the base of her neck extended up the right side of her head; that the back of her legs were sore; that she could not lie on the affected side, was worse resting, and that her feet and legs felt cold and were cold to touch. I ordered her Rhus Tox. 200c, three doses at twelve-hour intervals. Five weeks later she could report that the rheumatism was better.

These two remedies are the first to be thought of in a case of 'rheumatism', although individualisation may lead to the consideration of deeper-acting remedies. The next most frequently prescribed in my short series was Calcarea Carb. Charles Wheeler pointed out that the choice of Calcarea was determined by the general symptoms of constitution and temperament rather than the local symptoms in back and limbs.

General symptoms are the extreme susceptibility to cold, and therefore the Calcarea patient is the opposite to the Sulphur patient, who finds relief from cold and is aggravated by heat. Another general symptom is the profuse sweating of the head at night; a further symptom is slowness, bodily and mental, whereas in contrast Clarke points out that Sulphur is quick and active. In general appearance Calcarea patients are plump, with large heads and pale skins which can flush easily; this vasomotor instability is further illustrated by the tendency of the cold feet to get warm in bed and burn. Neatby and Stonham consider that Calcarea patients are blondes with blue eyes; in spite of the general plumpness, their necks tend to emaciate, and Kent says they have a tendency to alopecia areata; Hahnemann, after proving his special preparation of Calcarea Carb., and using it for many years, came to the conclusion that it was rarely if ever indicated in women whose menses appeared at the right time or later; in Calcarea subjects, the menses always appeared early.

As far as rheumatic pains are concerned they are most likely to be felt in parts on which the body has lain for a time, so it is not surprising that the worst time for Calcarea patients is 2–3 a.m. Kent does not recommend repetition of Calcarea in aged persons; Wheeler states it has a close relation to Rhus Tox., but that it is incompatible with Bryonia. Kent also asserts that taking a bath stops the action of Calcarea, but he does not say whether it is a hot or cold bath that matters.

A married lady of sixty, who twenty-five years before had been an active and energetic woman but who had now slowed down both bodily and mentally. She had put on weight and was easily tired by exertion. Her energetic and driving second husband expected her to accompany him on his sailing and fishing expeditions, and she often came home cold and exhausted after crewing for him or rowing him out to fish. She would wake up after a disturbed night, very stiff and aching, particularly in the back, the buttocks and the calves of the legs. I ordered a single dose of Calcarea Carb. 30c and did not hear from her again for seven months, when she telephoned me because she had contracted an acute sinusitis.

These three remedies, Bryonia, Rhus Tox. and Calcarea Carb., are the ones I have used most frequently in rheumatic conditions, but on occasion I have used ten other remedies in a one-year period.

There were another eight I have considered but did not use, as I decided in the end that they were not the simillimum for the particular patient involved. Of these I think first of Actaea Racemosa, also known as Cimicifuga; it is indicated in rheumatic disorders when associated with gynaecological complaints, and characterised by depression and loquacious grumbling; it is a cold remedy.

Colocynth has proved a valuable remedy in lumbago and sciatica, often associated with subluxations of the vertebral joints; it is useful after manipulation, especially in those patients with long backs when recurrence of the subluxation is frequent; it is another cold remedy, and the rheumatic pains are better for warmth and hard pressure. All my Colocynth patients were tall women, indignant and furious at stupid decisions enforced by their bosses.

Dulcamara is a remedy very susceptible to damp and wet. There is an allergic element in these patients, so that it resembles Rhus Tox. as it does in the restlessness, the pains being better for movement and worse for rest; I think the accompanying skin eruptions are characteristically either urticaria or warts.

Another Rhus-like patient in the restlessness, pains worse for keeping quiet, is Kali Iod., although it is the opposite of the cold shivering Rhus hugging the fire. The Kali Iod. patient cannot endure hot rooms, must be out in the open air, and does not get tired after walking like Rhus; the Kali Iod. patient is an individual of cruel temper, abusive with his wife and children. Another Kali salt is Kali Bichromicum, which was proved by the English homoeopath Drysdale. Characteristic features are that the pains shift about from spot to spot; spot is the operative word – the painful spot can be covered with the point of the finger. The pains appear and disappear suddenly. As well as these pains there are the restlessness and sleeplessness of Rhus. Kali Bich. appears to be best suited for fair-haired chubby persons.

Ledum is a remedy which like Bryonia is worse from movement; but the characteristic symptom is that in spite of the coldness all over, the pains are worse from the warmth of the bed, and relieved by cold applications, even sitting with the feet in cold water; in contrast, Rhus Tox. and Calc. Carb. are worse from bathing, especially from cold baths.

I have used the polychrests Lycopodium, Natrum Mur., Sepia, Silica and Sulphur when indicated on general and constitutional grounds, rather than on local symptoms.

The symptoms that differentiate Mercurius are the tremor, which is more pronounced than in any of the other rheumatic remedies. The sweating is as profuse as in Calc. Carb. and gives no relief. The

Mercurius patient is worse from sunset to sunrise; both cold and heat aggravate, indeed it is the change of temperature that is the precondition of pain developing.

Mezereum is another remedy to be thought of in rheumatic states. Hahnemann says it has proved useful in illnesses accompanied by moist eruptions of the scalp, inflammation of the eyes, chronic vaginal discharges and shortening of a lower limb; the body itches at night. It is one of the remedies like Ledum where the pains are worse from heat. The painful parts are numb; the apparent shortening of the lower limb is due to muscular contraction around the hip joint.

The pains of Phytolacca come and go suddenly like those of Kali Bich. They move about and change place, but unlike Kali Bich. they tend to radiate in various directions. Like Bryonia, the pains are worse on movement, like Rhus Tox., the Phytolacca patient is sensitive to damp weather and cold air. Other indications that would make me think of Phytolacca would be concomitant disorders of the mammary glands.

Another polychrest is Pulsatilla. This is a warm-blooded remedy, so that even in cold weather the patient goes about in light clothing. The general symptoms are the main indications; the joint and muscle pains tend to shift from place to place although not as suddenly as in Kali Bich. The pains are better for slow movement and cold applications – the opposite of Bryonia.

Lastly, let me refer to Ruta, which I have found the remedy of choice when bursae are involved. The Ruta patient is as restless as Rhus Tox. and as sensitive to cold damp weather. Ruta is especially suited to robust patients; if my rheumatic patients should complain at the same time of eye-strain or prolapse of the rectum, I would think of Ruta.

It is useful to think of sets of opposing remedies when the local modalities are strong. If moving the joint aggravates, think of Bryonia, Ledum and Phytolacca; if it ameliorates, consider Rhus Tox., Dulcamara, Kali Iod., Kali Bich., Pulsatilla and Ruta. Other modalities will differentiate between them, such as the aggravation from heat of Bryonia, Ledum, Kali Iod. and Mezereum.

If the joint is better from cold, think of Bryonia, Ledum and Pulsatilla; if worse, consider Rhus Tox., Calc. Carb., Mercurius, Phytolacca and Ruta.

The two remedies outstandingly worse for damp are Rhus Tox. and Dulcamara. Those which must be considered if dampness improves the joint (and the patient) are Causticum and Nux Vomica.

Chapter 11

Childhood Dyspepsia

The pictures of individual remedies are based not only on the original provings but also on the combined experiences of a series of homoeopathic physicians. They established the clinical value of these remedies when selected, not routinely, but according to individual symptoms and the constitutional makeup of their patients. I refer to the writings on materia medica of Hahnemann, Borland, John Henry Clarke, Hale, Hering, Richard Hughes, Kent, Neatby and Stonham, and Royal.

I have found the following three remedies useful when treating children suffering from gastro-intestinal disorders.

Cina

Its use as a vermifuge dates from the time of Hippocrates; but Kent advises his students to forget about the worms and to study the remedy as a whole in its action on the human mind and body. The active principle is santonin, a derivative of naphthalene; pharmacologists agree that it has a selective action on roundworms, the ascarides, but that it has little effect on the other intestinal parasites. They point out that poisoning with santonin may result in yellow vision, twitching of muscles, grinding of the teeth, nausea and vomiting.

Hahnemann proved Cina with the help of five assistants; he did not lay much stress on the digestive symptoms but pointed out the restlessness and the longing for many different things; the Cina patient refuses everything that is offered to him, even if it is what he likes best; the Cina child cannot be quieted by any persuasion and is insensible to caresses. Hahnemann's pupils Noack and Trinks drew attention to the clean tongue of Cina.

Hering emphasised the digestive symptoms: great hunger, even after eating, gnawing sensation in the stomach, pain felt above the umbilicus; with these pains, cold sweat on the forehead, a pale face, dark rings round the eyes, with a white ring round the mouth. The child grinds his teeth in his sleep, can even have hiccoughs while sleeping without waking up; he does not want to be touched, cannot bear anyone to come near him.

Clarke says the Cina patient is peevish and offended by the slightest thing.

Kent reminds us that though Cina has been thought of as a children's remedy, it is effective in adults if the indicating symptoms are present. He too comments on the touchiness both mental and physical; he speaks of the hyperaesthesia; the Cina child cannot have its hair combed or brushed; there is irritation of the nose; the child rubs his nose on the pillow, rubs and picks his nose; he prefers to sleep lying on his belly, and rolls his head when asleep; Kent underlines the hunger after eating, indeed even after vomiting. The stool is pale and the child smells sour; there is gurgling in the oesophagus when the child is swallowing, often very audible.

Neatby and Stonham call attention to the diarrhoea of thin, white, sour-smelling stools; they add that the typical white face can alternate with a red, hot face.

Finally, Borland makes the distinction between the Cina child and the Chamomilla child. Both are difficult to manage when they are ill; both want to be picked up and carried about; but he says the Cina child is more obstinate and stubborn, while the Chamomilla child is more unstable; he compares the Cina white watery stools with the copious green motions of Chamomilla.

Borland sees the Cina subject as a chilly person; he reminds us of the twitchings and the typical yawns; the Cina patient cannot see a joke, and is more likely to be ill in the summer and during dentition.

It is well to be reminded that one of the antidotes to Cina is peppermint, so often a constituent of toothpaste, sweets and chocolates. Camphor can act as an antidote; coffee too is an antidote for some remedies, but other subjects are actually better for it. I am not in favour of wholesale restriction of cosmetics, foods and drinks because of the theoretical possibilities of antidotal effects. I realise that some of the older authorities would consider this too permissive.

Case
An only child of eighteen months was brought to me; it had already been seen by a paediatrician at a teaching hospital who considered it a likely candidate for coeliac disease, although full investigations had been postponed for a year. This girl was a problem in the home. She slept very badly, keeping her parents walking about the bedroom all night; she was a very hungry child who never seemed to be satisfied; she vomited her

meals but still demanded to be fed. When I first saw her, she was a thin pale child with a twitch of the left eyelid; she rubbed her nose very hard; her mother reported that the child passed a pale watery stool but was very sensitive and made a great fuss when she cleaned her up.

I gave the child Cina 30c, to be repeated after each action of the bowels, and in less than ten days she was passing a normal stool and her appetite was no longer ravenous. Later, as a schoolgirl, she was inclined to digestive upsets, particularly in the summer months, but a dose of Cina 200c generally cleared these up quickly. Eventually, in adolescence, she outgrew both parents, had a very successful school and university career and now copes with a large dental practice.

Although this case has no direct reference to dyspepsia, I have had very satisfactory results in whooping cough with Cina in children of this temperament; it is worth remembering this alternative rather than to prescribe Drosera in a routine way.

I remember one boy of six, whose mother told me he ground his teeth in his sleep so loudly that she could hear him in the next-door bedroom. Unlike many pertussis cases he would not be held or supported in the whooping paroxysm; Cina controlled the paroxysms very quickly.

Graphites

When I first practised homoeopathy, my stereotype of Graphites was of a stout menopausal woman. After attending Dr Borland's lectures I realised that it was a remedy of much greater scope and had a sphere of action in children as well.

Graphites was a late introduction of Hahnemann's, and his provings first appeared in his *Chronic Diseases*. He called attention to the voracious hunger, the morning nausea, the eructations and belchings. The Victorian Hughes only saw it useful in chronic eczema; the typical eruption, he wrote, was the transformation of the primary vesicle into a crust from under which oozed a golden glutinous moisture.

The American Royal said that the successful prescription of Graphites depended on the recognition of the make-up of the patient, with the typical skin and mucous membrane; a fleshy subject who had suddenly increased in weight, with poor circulation, was more likely to benefit from Graphites. Clarke speaks of the rough hard skin. Borland contrasts the rough hard skin with the soft sweaty skin of Calc. Carb., who was also likely to be fat.

Neatby and Stonham describe the Graphites patient as chilly and sensitive to cold, yet wanting to be in the open air, uncomfortable in a warm room and in a warm bed; they have a hunger pain one hour after eating and are better for hot drinks; they are constipated, passing a large hard stool that is often covered with stringy mucus. The Graphites patient, they say, tends to have fissures and cracks in the skin, round the corners of the mouth and on the eyelids, behind the ears; the nails are brittle and deformed.

Borland, too, says that the Graphites child develops cracks in the skin in cold weather; they are fat, pale, chilly children, who flush under stress and are liable to nosebleeds; easily tired, they are bad travellers; they have big appetites but curiously have an aversion to sweets and have a marked dislike of fish.

They do not show signs of allergy. Borland's experience was that Graphites children were timid and lazy and tried to avoid school work; he compared them with Petroleum children, who also had a skin with a tendency to crack and chap; who were also bad travellers, car-sick and sea-sick; but the Petroleum child was usually thin, in contrast to the fat Graphites child.

Case

A girl aged eight was the daughter of a very overweight mother. A plump constipated child who had a stool every third day; she had a hearty appetite; her mother was worried about her pallor and her apathy about school, though the girl had been tested and was of superior intelligence. She had had attacks of nose bleeding; she had crusts on the eyelids; and was liable to attacks of abdominal pain, which she used as an excuse to stay home from school.

She has made satisfactory improvement on Graphites; her school work has improved and she is progressing well.

Podophyllum

This remedy was a relatively late introduction to the pharmacopoeia by the American homoeopath Hale. It had been well known as a folk remedy to the American Indians before the discovery of America by the Europeans.

Hale called attention to the sallow skin and the tendency to prolapse of the rectum. Royal, a generation later, refers to the nausea, the colic in the early morning followed by the profuse offensive stools and the tendency to prolapse of the rectum. He felt that this gastro-enteritis was more likely to recur in hot weather.

J. H. Clarke says that the profuse diarrhoea can occur while the child is being bathed; he says the gushing diarrhoea can be painless and that there is a thirst for cold water; like Cina, the patient tends to grind the teeth and press the gums together.

Kent says Podophyllum is rarely indicated if the stool is not offensive. Borland underlines the offensiveness of the motion; the odour penetrates the whole house; the stool is very profuse, being passed with a good deal of flatus and gurgling in the intestines and resulting in prolapse of the rectum. Before the action of the bowels, most probably early in the morning, there is intense colic, with some relief from heat and pressure; there is nausea and vomiting of bile-stained material; the tongue is thickly-coated yellow, as if mustard had been spread on it; the child looks dehydrated, pale with sunken eyes. Often the history is of a previous meal of stewed fruit and cream. I find a sizeable proportion of summer gastroenteritis cases respond satisfactorily to this remedy.

Case

A rather stolid little boy of four with a very tough young father and a very dependent inadequate mother; an overactive child who nevertheless sleeps well at night but is liable, as indeed were all the family, to alimentary infections. He stands hot weather badly; is liable to attacks of colic, becomes pale and refuses food because of nausea, develops severe colic, and then passes profuse offensive stools, so profuse that his doting grandmother wonders where it all comes from. I have doubts about the hygiene in this house, but since the mother and the grandmother have been instructed in the indications for Podophyllum I have heard much less frequently from them about this little boy.

Chapter 12

Haemorrhoids

About 1100 B.C., in the Eastern Mediterranean, an epidemic of piles broke out among the Philistines. Many died and the survivors suffered great distress from a plague of 'emerods', as the Jacobean bishops so termed them. Was this a fulminating dysentery complicated by prolapsed haemorrhoids? Had some of the food at a celebratory banquet been a bit off?

Even in Hahnemann's time there were no effective remedies for haemorrhoids. When he published the two volumes of his *Materia Medica* they included sixty-seven remedies and a total of over thirty-three thousand symptoms. Of all those thousands of symptoms, only forty-eight referred directly to haemorrhoids, a total of just over one-tenth of one per cent. In his foreword to the Sulphur provings, Hahnemann states that some orthodox physicians claimed to have cured some haemorrhoidal affections with Sulphur, but of course had used far too large doses. Only twenty-three of Hahnemann's remedies had symptoms referring to haemorrhoids, and of these only half a dozen had more than two symptoms each. They were: Pulsatilla (10), Arsenicum (4), Ignatia (4), Nux Vomica (4), Chamomilla (3) and Ferrum (3).

Hughes in his *Manual of Therapeutics* comments on the virtues of Sulphur and Nux Vomica in the treatment of haemorrhoids. He recommends they should be given in alternation and states that they act better thus than when either is given separately. The Ignatia patient suffers from haemorrhoids that prolapse with every stool and have to be replaced; sharp 'stitches' shoot up the rectum. Of course, the characteristic Ignatia temperament must be present. It is curious that a hundred years ago Hering thought there were many more Ignatia persons in North America than Nux Vomica persons. Was immigration the explanation?

Paeonia is a remedy known to the ancients and included by Dioscorides in his *Materia Medica*. There is intolerable pain in the rectum, during and after stool, oozing of moisture from the rectum and intense chilliness after stool. A feature of the Paeonia patient is terrifying dreams and nightmares.

Verbascum was proved by Hahnemann. (The plant was known to the English herbalist Gerard.) Clarke only found it useful as an external application to relieve the itching of haemorrhoids in the form of an ointment.

The breakthrough in the treatment of haemorrhoids happened not in Europe but across the Atlantic, some years after Hahnemann's death. Dr E. M. Hale reported that after many years of experience of using the sixty-odd remedies then in the materia medica, he found that although their range of action was very wide, they did not cover many symptoms, or indeed many illnesses. In North America, remarkable cures had been brought to his notice by indigenous remedies in the hands of eclectic and domestic practitioners. ('Eclectic practitioners' were doctors who used homoeopathic remedies without committing themselves to membership of homoeopathic societies, and 'domestic practitioners' were simply ordinary people using folk medicine.) For several years he collected everything that had been published concerning the indigenous plants, including all the clinical and theoretical information, that his colleagues could provide, adding to this his own provings and researches. In 1864 he published in Detroit his *New Remedies*, which added forty-four drugs to the pharmacopoeia. These included such essential remedies as Arum, Baptisia, Caulophyllum, Cimicifuga, Eupatorium, Gelsemium, Hydrastis, Phytolacca, Podophyllum, Rumex and Sanguinaria. Besides these indispensable remedies there are three others which have an almost specific effect on the rectum and anus: these are Hamamelis, Aesculus, and Collinsonia.

First of all there is *Hamamelis virginica*, the witchhazel. It was the famous Tradescant family who in the early 18th century had a monopoly of plant introductions from America into England and were responsible for planting witchhazel in Britain; but it was in America that Mr Pond produced his world famous extract, and Mr Pond's doctor was the famous Constantine Hering, a favourite pupil of Hahnemann. Pond told his doctor what the extract was made of, and Hering at once organised tests for claims made for the extract. He found it was useful in the chronic effects from mechanical injuries and painful and bleeding haemorrhoids. Hale then devotes fifteen pages of his book to case records from eighteen different doctors.

Richard Hughes was quick to appreciate the value of Hamamelis. Within a couple of years of the publication of Hale's book he was reporting in the *British Homoeopathic Journal* a successful cure with that remedy. He says in his book, 'I have cured case after case of bleeding piles with Hamamelis and never failed in seventeen years. I would never be without it in my pocket case.' He used the 1x, 1c or 2c potencies. He thought it was better than Pulsatilla in phlebitis, but did not recommend it for phlegmasia alba dolens, the 'white leg' that sometimes follows childbirth.

Another enthusiast for Hamamelis was Dr Compton Burnett, father of the famous novelist Ivy Compton Burnett and uncle of Dr Margery Blackie. He wrote what he called 'a little treatise' – *Diseases of the Veins* – and Hamamelis was the easy winner of some fifty remedies that he included. He also noted that many Hamamelis patients complained that 'my back feels as if it would break off'.

Are bleeding piles to be the main indication for Hamamelis? That would be pathological prescribing with a vengeance. It was in fact the principle that Richard Hughes was so industrious in preaching; but in his chapter on Hamamelis he points out that it was not properly proved for another twenty years after its introduction to the homoeopaths. He also recommends it for simple phlebitis and in varicose veins, saying that it is more suitable when the state of the vessels is the cause of the haemorrhage rather than the condition of the blood. He adds that the other locale of action of Hamamelis is the sexual organs, quoting the case of an American prover who suffered so severely from neuralgia in the testes that he had to discontinue the proving.

Clarke emphasises the intense soreness of the parts that are bleeding, in contrast to those where passive haemorrhages are painless. This soreness is a feature of the rheumatic pains that occur as side effects when low potencies of Hamamelis are given for varicose veins.

Hamamelis patients are sensitive to the open air and rainy weather. It is the remedy of choice for the absorption of intraocular haemorrhages, better than either Arnica or Calendula. Kent claims the shed blood is dark, and that bright red blood is the exception. Varicose veins are much worse in pregnancy, indeed so much so that the woman can neither walk nor stand. While Pond's extract was made from the leaves, Hale used the bark of the Hamamelis shrub for the homoeopathic remedy.

The horse chestnut, *Aesculus*, was originally used in veterinary medicine. The Turks ground the chestnuts into a coarse flour which was given to horses that were broken-winded. Normally animals do not touch them. The Austrian ambassador at Constantinople sent conkers to Vienna. Some authorities say the horse chestnut is a native of Northern Greece, others favour the Balkans. In Elizabethan times it was described as a rare foreign tree, but by the time of Charles I, John Tradescant had a chestnut tree which he brought back from Italy growing in his garden at South Lambeth. Although the tree is not indigenous to the United States it was naturalised there, and the fruit was used in a proving by American doctors. Hale included it in his *New Remedies.*

Hahnemann dismissed Aesculus, commenting that the sole symptom it produces is a constrictive feeling in the chest and that it would be found useful in asthma; but he was speaking of the bark, which in Europe had been used as a substitute for Cinchona. Hale reports in detail provings of Aesculus by six doctors. One of them, Dr Burt, commented, 'Not one of our remedies produced so many and so strongly marked symptoms of haemorrhoids as the Aesculus.'

Hughes, reviewing Hale's book, writes that his experience with Aesculus in haemorrhoids had been very satisfactory; there is little tendency to haemorrhage but much sense of bearing down and fullness with constipation. He quotes an illustrative case of a woman with a thirty-five year history of haemorrhoids who was liable to attacks of very dreadful pain. She could not sit, stand or lie; the only possible position was kneeling; the pain was like a knife sawing backwards and forwards – a martyrdom of agony. She took various homoeopathic remedies with no relief. At last she consulted Dr Hughes, who ordered her Aesculus 2c, three drops in water, night and morning. At the end of a month she was wonderfully better, the bowels acted much more freely and the protrusion of the haemorrhoidal mass became softer.

Hughes was sceptical about the headache and backache reported by Burt in his personal proving, because these symptoms turned up in his provings of seven other remedies, and Hughes considered them peculiarities of the heroic doctor's constitution. Burnett did not agree with Hale that Aesculus was not indicated if the patient was constipated. His extensive experience led him to say that it is indicated very strongly when the patient is constipated. Additional symptoms he quotes are throbbing in the abdominal and pelvic cavities, dull backache, and purple-coloured haemorrhoids.

Burnett throws out 'clinical chips', as he phrases it, from his own workshop, quoting some very severe cases where the rectum and haemorrhoids are prolapsed, almost strangulated. He recommends external treatment combined with internal treatment. Externally, lint soaked in Hamamelis mother tincture is applied to the haemorrhoidal mass when the patient goes to bed, and is left in position all night. The next night it is replaced with a fresh piece of saturated lint, all aperients being absolutely forbidden. If the patient would not agree to this prohibition Dr Burnett invariably declined to take on the case.

Of almost equal importance, the patient was forbidden to defaecate until he positively could not hold out any longer. The reason is that these patients often have a habit of pressing at stool like a pregnant woman in labour, and the pressure from above will do more harm than the doctor can repair.

Clarke says that Aesculus patients as a rule are despondent and irritable, very much worse for walking: Kent defines this aggravation from walking as a pain through the sacrum into the hips. Allen says the Aesculus patient is miserably cross – the rectum feels as if full of small sticks, and after defaecation there is intense pain in the anus for hours.

The third haemorrhoidal remedy from America is Collinsonia. In the mountains and hills of Virginia, Kentucky and Georgia, it was considered a panacea by the common people and used much as the common people in Germany used Arnica. Doctors found it invaluable in cases of habitual constipation, producing not just transient relief but correcting in a permanent manner the disorder of the digestive system. Another doctor, referring to his own case, reported that after suffering for fifteen years from the reactive effects of a series of powerful aperients administered systematically during his infancy, after a month's use of Collinsonia had cured himself and had no need to repeat it in the following year.

Fowler quotes the case of a man suffering from haemorrhoids that had made his life almost a burden and completely disabled him from business. The infusion of the chopped root acted as an emetic, but a smaller dose resulted in a cure in three weeks. This patient had been a victim of the most resolute constipation and never had relief without the aid of enemas. As these could not be administered without irritation and pain, they could not be tolerated more often than every fourth or fifth day. The remedy established a free and natural daily action of the bowels.

Hughes does not refer to Collinsonia when he reviewed Hale's *New Remedies*, but in the second edition he found a short proving. He had the greatest confidence in this remedy for constipation and haemorrhoids in the middle and latter months of pregnancy. He wrote, 'It may be resorted to with advantage whenever Aesculus fails. Where the haemorrhoids date from pregnancy or labour and the condition has become chronic, there is no remedy to compare with it for efficacy.' Hughes nearly always used the 2x potency.

Clarke compares Aesculus and Collinsonia – Aesculus has a sense of fullness in the rectum which Collinsonia does not have. As a rule

Aesculus piles do not bleed, whereas those of Collinsonia bleed persistently. Aesculus has pain, soreness and aching in the back, worse by walking. Collinsonia has more persistent constipation with colic. Aesculus may be constipated. Collinsonia should not be used in low potencies if the patient has organic heart disease; Allen nevertheless recommends that it should be considered in heart disease complicated with haemorrhoids. He says that the slightest mental emotion or excitement aggravates the symptoms.

Lastly, I must mention Aloes, included by Compton Burnett in his little book. This remedy has a typical diarrhoea; has to hurry to the lavatory immediately after eating and drinking; is driven out of bed early in the morning to defaecate; the tender hot sore haemorrhoids are relieved by cold water. The Aloes patient is worse in hot, dry weather.

I would expect the three American remedies, Hamamelis, Aesculus and Collinsonia, to cover more than 80% of your cases of haemorrhoids.

Chapter 13

Asthma

It has been estimated that one per cent of the population are liable to asthma and that it is most common at the age of six. In most of the cases there is an allergic family history and it is common to hear of the baby with infantile eczema, developing so-called bronchitis at the toddler stage, and asthma becoming the diagnosis when he reaches infant school.

The Japanese research worker Ishizaka was the first to demonstrate that the immunoglobulin IgE was the antibody responsible for atopic sensitivity. Besides paediatricians and physicians, psychiatrists and psychologists have also been interesting themselves in asthma. Psychiatrists agree that there is no specific personality type predisposed to asthma; this would confirm the experience of homoeopaths who see good results from remedies such as Pulsatilla and Phosphorus, whose characteristic mental symptomatologies are widely different.

Asthmatic children do appear to be handicapped by the attitudes of their parents, who are statistically three times more often over-anxious and over-protective than the parents of normal children.

Psychiatrists have been investigating the effects of hypnosis in asthma, but preliminary results in a controlled trial were not very impressive, and critics have pointed out that it is possible to suggest successfully that there would be freedom from wheezing without any improvement in respiratory function, and that sticky mucous plugs throughout the lungs could not be removed by suggestion. However, subsequent experience has shown that hypnosis does have a part to play in treatment.

Orthodox physicians claim that there are three ways of treating asthma: (1) by avoiding the causative allergen if known, (2) by desensitisation, and (3) by drug therapy. The allergen is difficult to identify, multiple allergens are frequent, and precipitation of an attack might be the result of emotional and/or physical stresses as well as exposure to the allergen. Desensitisation could improve but not cure four out of five asthmatics, but this only lasts six months. The majority of asthmatics referred to homoeopathic doctors have already had orthodox drug therapy, and this at once raises serious problems. One homoeopath has pointed out how steroid therapy masks the symptomatology, and worse still, results in lack of reactivity to homoeopathic remedies.

To identify the best indications for the homoeopathic remedy and ensure a satisfactory response, it would seem desirable to wean the patient from steroids, since these cloud modalities. This is not without serious risks, and it has been shown that asthmatics are particularly vulnerable to rebound phenomena after withdrawal of their steroids: twenty per cent in one series developed status asthmaticus, and there was a high mortality. My own experience confirms this danger. A patient aged sixty was referred to me by a Glasgow consultant. She had been warned that if homoeopathic treatment were to succeed she would have to discontinue steroid treatment. Without waiting to see me she had stopped her prednisone, and when I called on her I found her in status asthmaticus. I had no alternative but to refer her at once to hospital for intensive life-saving therapy. A second patient, aged sixty-eight, a non-allergic asthmatic, was on prednisone twice a day and tranquillisers. I suggested he reduced his prednisone to once a day and ordered him Kali Carb. 30c. In three weeks he was improved but two weeks later relapsed, and his family doctor had to give him three times the original dose of prednisone to control the asthma.

During the late 1960s there was a rise in the death rate from asthma, and this increase was most noticeable in children over ten. Research showed that the death rate in the age range 10–14 had increased seven times in seven years. Suspicion fell on the aerosol inhalers using isoprenaline, and reduction in the use of these inhalers was followed by a drop in mortality. In any case it was shown that aerosol bronchodilators were only effective in the milder attacks of asthma with forced expiratory ventilation in the range 55–69%. While antihistamines have been useful in allergic complaints such as hay fever and urticaria, they are of little help in asthma. Even aminophylline can produce adverse reactions, particularly in women over sixty.

One of the latest treatments for asthma is insufflation of sodium cromoglycate from a special spinhaler. However, this drug must be looked on with some suspicion by homoeopaths, as its rationale is to inhibit the effect of certain antigen/antibody reactions. This could lead to patients being less responsive to homoeopathic remedies – the same disadvantage as treatment with steroid preparations.

This résumé of the orthodox treatment of asthma points to the desirability of early homoeopathic treatment of the asthmatic while still a very young child. Steroid or cromoglycate treatment interferes with the natural defence mechanisms by which homoeopathic remedies may act, for allergy and immunity are indissolubly related.

In the treatment of asthma there are two problems. Firstly the treatment of the acute attack, and secondly the prevention of further attacks by constitutional treatment. Probably the most commonly indicated remedy in the acute attack, especially in children, is Ipecacuanha. The bad cold that ends in chest trouble in infants is often asthma – the symptoms have a rapid onset, the child is pale, looks very anxious, the breathing is laboured, and there is a coarse rattling respiration. In adult asthmatics, Ipecacuanha will give relief when the attack has been precipitated by cold damp weather.

The other acute remedy that I have found valuable is Arsenicum Album. The patient is very anxious, afraid he is going to die, restless; if able to climb out of bed he sits in a chair, keeps moving from one place to another; at last becomes so weak that he is no longer able to move, and lies in extreme prostration. He wants to be covered warmly, hovers around the radiator, suffers from draughts. The asthma comes on at midnight or after, then he coughs dry and wheezing, and needs to sit up and hold his chest.

Both these asthmatic types are chilly mortals, but there is also a warm asthmatic. He is worse in a hot room and better in the open air – the characteristic Pulsatilla patient. Pulsatilla was one of the first remedies proved by Hahnemann, which he described with indications as to the temperamental type: timid, tearful, mild, yielding and slow, with changeable moods. It is not indicated for persons who make quick decisions. It is a remedy often indicated at puberty. Patients of the Pulsatilla type crave open air, dislike warmth and stuffy rooms, and are better for movement. The asthma comes on in the late afternoon and evening.

A child patient aged fourteen had a two-year history of asthma, a previous history of eczema and hay fever, and had been treated for amoebic dysentery with emetine. An ear, nose and throat specialist had carried out an antral puncture. Examination showed enlarged pale turbinates. She had no further attacks for two years after one dose of Pulsatilla 1M.

Once the attack has been controlled, treatment to prevent further attacks must be organised on constitutional lines. In established cases of asthma, especially in adults, it may take one to two years to control.

A patient aged fifty-five who consulted me had a long history of asthma. She had begun prednisone but had been warned off it by her sister, the matron of a private nursing home. She had an initial dose of the nosode Psorinum; two months later a dose of Apis. Her chest symptoms improved but she had a reaction in her nasal sinuses. This reaction cleared up after Silica, and twenty-seven months later she was free of attacks. She had no further attacks in the following two years.

The other asthmatic remedy-types besides Pulsatilla which are worse off in a warm room are Chamomilla, Iodum and Spongia. Chamomilla is a bad-tempered, angry subject not afraid to die, indeed would rather die than put up with suffering. Anger can bring on an attack. It is not indicated in patients who bear their symptoms patiently and with resignation.

Iodum also cannot stand heat, but in constrast to the blonde, plump Pulsatilla, Iodum is a scrawny brunette with dark hair and tawny skin. She is always anxious, in a hurry and must keep moving. She is hungry and thirsty, whereas Pulsatilla is anxious and thirstless.

My experience with Spongia is that when indicated, the patient has always had some cardiac complication as well as the tendency to asthma. The Spongia type is characteristically a blue-eyed blonde with an enlarged heart. The asthma attack wakes the patient out of sleep after midnight. In spite of wanting cool air, the Spongia patient is better for warm drinks and warm food.

Some of the acute Arsenicum types will continue to improve on Arsenicum in the intervals, but others will require other remedies to clear up their case.

The patient responding to Dulcamara (the woody nightshade) is very sensitive to weather changes, particularly changes to cold and damp, and is liable to asthma in the autumn. Dulcamara has various skin eruptions and a tendency to warts.

Natrum Sulph. is another remedy very sensitive to damp. The asthma is worse in wet weather. Diarrhoea is quite a frequent accompaniment to the asthmatic attack – the attacks being most likely to occur between 6–9 p.m. Natrum Sulph. patients are depressed and have suicidal thoughts. The Natrum Sulph. asthmatic is not restless like the Arsenicum patient, but is better for keeping still.

The Sambucus patient is worse for cold air, but like Spongia sleeps into the attack of asthma. He does not perspire when asleep but breaks into a perspiration on waking.

The Kali Carb. patient will be an adult. I have never seen it indicated in a child and have generally had the best results in the elderly. Kali Carb. patients tend to be dark-haired, over-weight, with characteristic water-bags between the eyebrow and upper eyelid. The asthmatic attack tends to come on between 3–4 a.m. The patient gets relief sitting bent forward with the elbows propped upon a bed-table. The Kali Carb. asthmatic is full of fear, cannot bear to be left alone and yet is very irritable. They are very ticklish and cannot bear to be touched.

One of the most important of the chilly asthmatic remedies is Phosphorus. Phosphorus patients tend to be tall, slender, fair or red-haired – the hair is fine and soft. They are quick in thinking and lively in action. They too are afraid when alone, afraid of the dark – afraid of thunderstorms. They feel better coming into a warm room. Unlike Sambucus and Spongia, the Phosphorus patient is generally better after sleep. The Phosphorus patient prefers cold drinks, in contrast to the Spongia patient, who will choose warm drinks.

There are, however, patients who do not at first respond to these usual remedies and may require one of the nosodes. If the first attack of asthma followed a measles infection, a dose of Morbillinum may clear up the case. Psorinum is useful when there is an alternation between hay fever and asthma. It is one of the chilly remedies, and the Psorinum patient generally gives the impression of being overclothed, if an adult. Overanxious mothers also tend to overclothe their asthmatic children.

In any allergic case it is important to avoid sensitising the patient to the homoeopathic remedy, and this means using a single dose at a time, not repeating until the good effect seems to have been exhausted. In treating allergic patients I usually start with a single dose of the 30th potency and gradually work up through the 200th to the 1000th. I do not go below the 30th or above the 1000th potency.

Chapter 14

Hay Fever

Hay fever usually shows itself in the early teens, but some potential hay fever subjects develop seasonal conjunctivitis two or three years before puberty; I have also seen this seasonal conjunctivitis in an adult polo player without accompanying rhinorrhoea. As well as the seasonal hay fevers, there is the group of patients who suffer from non-allergic rhinitis.

Patients with non-seasonal types of rhinorrhoea turn up in our surgeries often labelling themselves as 'chronic catarrh' or 'sinusitis'. Their symptoms may be due to animal contacts – cats, dogs, budgerigars or the ponies beloved of the small girl devotees. Then there are the occupational series of furriers, woodworkers and florists, not to forget people exposed to feathers in bedmaking and to dust mites in cleaning the house.

Another group of non-seasonal rhinitises are associated with disorders of the thermostatic apparatus. Rhinitis is provoked by sudden changes of temperature – I had one patient who developed 'hay fever' each time she was out in a snowstorm. Allied to this group are the menopausal and post-menopausal women whose sneezing bouts accompany hot flushes, or else substitute for them.

The three main complications of hay fever are sinusitis, polyps and asthma. I have not been helped much by X-rays, and have found skin tests misleading. So many of my hay fever patients appear to be sensitive to a very wide range of allergens.

The orthodox treatment of hay fever is by antihistamines, and in the majority of patients the treatment has to be continued indefinitely; desensitisation in pollen hypersensitivity involves a tedious series of injections which have to be repeated each year.

For students, the hay fever season coincides with examination dates. It is bad enough to try to write an examination paper handicapped by running eyes and nose and explosive sneezing, but the situation is made worse by the drowsiness that follows the use of antihistamines. One of my colleagues turned up for his viva in pharmacology with running eyes and nose, exploding with sneezes. He apologised to his examiner, who remarked, 'How very interesting', and proceeded to quiz him on the medical treatment of hay fever, the only aspect of pharmacology with which my colleague was really familiar.

It has been observed in asthma that different remedies are usually required for the acute attack than those required for the prevention between attacks. In my experience this holds good for hay fever too.

The remedy for acute hay fever is Arsenicum Album, which was one of the original remedies proved by Hahnemann. He was familiar with arsenic, as he had published a book on the forensic detection of arsenic poisoning in 1786, some years before his *Essay on a New Principle*. Hahnemann's tests for arsenic were a great improvement on former tests and were accurate in very high dilutions of the substance.

Features of the Arsenicum drug picture are: anxiety, restlessness, prostration, acrid discharges, thirst for frequent small quantities, and aggravation after midnight.

The Arsenicum patient is better in wet weather and worse in dry weather, as would be expected in any case of hay fever when pollen grains would be washed down by the rain. Royal emphasises the profuse watery discharges; he says the hay fever is worse in the open air, but again this is only to be expected. He says the Arsenicum hay fever has no relief from sneezing, the nose feels stopped up and the eyes water. Clarke says Arsenicum is the horse's remedy, Pulsatilla the sheep's remedy, and Antimony the pig's. He says the horse typifies the Arsenicum temperament: 'The horse is an exceedingly nervous animal, constantly moving about, restless to a degree, and very prone to take fright – quite a picture of the Arsenicum temperament.' Tyler says of the Arsenicum patient that he is so particular; she reminds us of how chilly he is, preferring hot drinks to cold, and indeed becoming ill after eating ices.

There are three remedies which I have found valuable in the constitutional treatment of this condition. I avoid giving the constitutional remedy in the hay fever season, and for the seasonal cases I usually ask the patient to take the treatment not later than the last week in February.

The first remedy is Apis. Bee venom was proved in America in 1835. The relevant symptoms in the proving of Apis are congestion of head and face, puffiness around eyes, lachrymation, photophobia, hot tears, and the nose swollen, red and oedematous.

Gross pointed out that Apis patients were worse in a warm room and better in the open air; they were worse for hot food and hot drinks; they preferred to wash in cold water. Royal stressed that they were thirstless. He compared them with Arsenicum patients, who were thirsty, wanted to be warm, and who had irritable alimentary tracts, whereas Apis patients had few digestive symptoms. Apis patients, he said, passed very scanty urine and often had renal complications. I have found Apis almost specific for angioneurotic oedema.

A patient in her early fifties had suffered from hay fever as a young woman, but had been free for several years. While on holiday in Switzerland she had been involved in a motor accident and suffered injuries to her rib-cage. On her return home, she found to her surprise that she could no longer pet the family cat without bringing on hay fever, at the same time developing angioneurotic oedema. I ordered her a single dose of Apis 30c. A month later she reported that she could now stroke the cat again without producing symptoms.

Another constitutional remedy is Petroleum. This was a remedy proved by Hahnemann, but has perhaps been rather neglected.

Gross says the Petroleum patient is better indoors and worse out of doors, which is what we should expect of the hay fever patient; he adds that the Petroleum patient is worse before a thunderstorm, worse from bright light and worse for smoking. Clarke says Petroleum patients are generally lean and slender persons with light hair and skin; their skin is extremely sensitive to contact with clothing, and there is a tendency to form cracks at mucocutaneous junctions. Their hair falls out, they are worse in winter, they become angry over trifles and their symptoms can be brought on by vexation.

However, the following example is interesting. A patient aged forty suffered from a non-seasonal rhinorrhoea and was one of the thermo-labile types; she was well in the summer, but when the frosts began in the autumn she used to wake up with a prickling in the nose and sneezed every cold morning. She had quite violent sneezing attacks during a snowstorm. On examination I noticed cracks between the alae nasi and the lips. She felt the cold; in the consulting room she removed in stages her headscarf, mufflers and neckscarf. The cracked nostrils made me think of Petroleum and her other symptoms were covered in the repertory. I ordered Petroleum 30c, one dose. She reported back at Easter and at midsummer. Beyond the odd sneeze her constant nasal drip had cleared up and the cracks in the nostril had healed. She had no rhinorrhoea the following winter.

The last remedy to consider is Psorinum. Psorinum was the first of the nosodes, being prepared from the sero-purulent matter from a scabies vesicle. Clarke writes that Psorinum patients are very chilly; they are restless persons and easily startled; they are reported to emit a disagreeable odour. Borland says Psorinum children are pale, delicate, peevish; they sweat on the least exertion, their faces are greasy; mental symptoms are hopelessness and despair of recovery. Neatby and Stonham comment on the coarse, scaly skin which itches in a warm bed and under warm clothing; the offensive perspiration occurs particularly on the palms of the hands and perineum. They are hungry people, especially in the night, getting out of bed in the small hours to forage in the larder.

Clarke cured more cases of hay fever with Psorinum than with any other single remedy. Borland confirms this; he says Psorinum is much the most commonly curative remedy given before the start of the hay fever season. He had never seen it help in the acute condition. I can confirm that Psorinum has been successful in the majority of my cases of hay fever when given at the end of February.

A patient in her late thirties, a dress designer and a keen gardener in her spare time, was liable to disabling hay fever each early summer. She was a thin, spare woman, very pessimistic that any improvement was possible; she had been through all the rigmarole of skin tests and her biggest reaction was to grass pollen. She had a pale face and dry hair and was very sensitive to cold; in the acute attack of hay fever she had intense photophobia and pulled the blinds down in any room where she was trying to work. She had a dose of Psorinum 30c in February following the first summer that I saw her; she had no further hay fever in the next thirty years.

I have not noticed the offensive odours that other homoeopathic writers have emphasised, in the considerable number of my adult hay fever patients. Some of my Psorinum patients have reacted to the first dose with urticaria, which did not persist.

Chapter 15

Miscellaneous Disorders

There are patients whose orthodox practitioner will have told them: 'There is nothing more I can do for you', 'You must learn to live with it', or 'I have used up all the shots in my locker'. Although these complaints are rarely fatal, and very often not even dangerous, they are often quite disabling and sufficiently severe to interfere with the patient's occupation and social and domestic life.

This chapter considers some of these conditions and the part that homoeopathic medicine can play in their relief.

Menière's Syndrome

A clergyman, now seventy years old, had been under orthodox treatment for some twelve years. He wrote that his doctor could offer no prospect of a cure and had agreed to another opinion. The doctor wrote to me, saying that his patient was averaging one attack a week in spite of treatment with barbiturates and tranquillisers. Five years earlier the patient had had a coronary thrombosis. The clergyman was a vigorous old gentleman of small physique who had served in the First World War. The attacks were sudden; he had fallen down on several occasions, was nauseated and had vomited on occasions. He had had attacks in church when in the pulpit, and had reluctantly resigned. He was deaf in the left ear, and between attacks there was a continuous tinnitus. After the attack, a headache lasted some two hours.

On examination, his blood pressure was 140/110, retinal arteries were contracted, venous crossings prominent. The left membrana tympani was indrawn, pale and atrophic. He was showing nerve deafness in the left ear, whereas hearing in the right ear was fair, although there was evidence of some impairment. There was nystagmus on looking to the right. He said that the tranquilliser had upset his vision and that he had discontinued it.

In the five months before he started homoeopathic treatment he had experienced eleven attacks of vertigo. He began treatment with a single dose of Cocculus 30c. Three months later he had one slight attack, and a further dose of Cocculus was prescribed. Nine months later he felt sufficiently confident to do a late Sunday duty for a fellow cleric, and after three further months could report a year without an attack. He kept in touch with me regularly. Two years later he wrote to say he had had no further attacks, that he had taken over a hundred services in twenty different churches, was planning to take three services each Sunday during the holiday months, and in addition was doing quite a lot of gardening, as well as all sorts of odd jobs and improvements in and around his bungalow.

The next case of Menière's syndrome illustrates some of the difficulties facing the homoeopathic physician who accepts a patient who has had much previous allopathic treatment.

Mr P. C., aged sixty-eight and retired, was a tall well-built man who had seen four specialists within ten years. His illness began with deafness in one ear and was later followed by attacks of vertigo, which had occurred when hedge clipping, standing in church, leaning back in his chair or watching television. He had vomited with these attacks and now noticed he was becoming more deaf in the right ear. He also suffered from asthma. As a result of his various consultations he was taking three vasodilator tablets a day, an antihistamine to deal with the sickness, three muscle relaxants a day, and an antihistamine tablet at night. He had a fine physique and his blood pressure was only 120/80.

I ordered him a single dose of Cocculus 30c and suggested that he should begin by discontinuing the vasodilator tablets in view of his low blood pressure. A month later he reported that the attacks were less frequent and less prolonged and that the hearing in his deaf ear had improved. In another two months he had had one attack of Menière's syndrome but had resumed his gardening activities. He accepted my suggestion to discard the muscle relaxants. In a further two months he had had one slight attack, could hear the hymns in church, and the tinnitus had altered, being now just a throbbing. A further dose of Cocculus was prescribed. In another two months he reported further improvement in his hearing. Over the next four months he made steady progress on one more dose of Cocculus and was able to attend concerts and operas with pleasure, without using a hearing aid.

Migraine
While not a dangerous disease, migraine can be very crippling. Miss B. G., fifty-eight, a tall grey-haired spinster, was housekeeper to a wealthy octogenarian who entertained on a large scale. Her attacks,

when she consulted me, were occurring once a week and laid her out for two days at a time. The attacks were usually right-sided. Her general practitioner had dieted her, but the only result was that the nausea accompanying the headache no longer ended in vomiting of bile. She complained of appalling depression and loss of memory accompanying the headaches. She said she had learned to control her temper in coping with the demands of her exigent employer.

She was given a single dose of Phosphorus 30c and went away for her annual holiday that summer. A month later she reported that though she had had an attack each week, the attacks were mild, and it was the first holiday for five years which she had not spent mostly in bed. Another dose of Phosphorus 30c was prescribed. In the next six weeks, she had only two attacks. She had a single dose of Phosphorus 30c at monthly intervals for the next three months, during which time she had three slight attacks but got over them quickly. She volunteered that she could not remember feeling as calm or contented before. Over the next six months she had only two slight attacks, after which she had another single dose of Phosphorus 30c. Within the next three months she had one fairly severe attack after the strain of entertaining a big house-party. At the end of ten months she looked a different person, had put on weight, was much less depressed – and felt very fit physically. She said she had never felt so peaceful.

Mrs V. M., aged forty-three, married, one child, was sent to me by her doctor for severe disabling headaches which had persisted for twelve years following the birth of her only child. The headache was always associated with the menstrual period; she usually woke with the headache, which was mostly right-sided and lasted all day, terminating in profuse vomiting of bile. She was exhausted the next day and unable to work at her part-time job as a tailoress. In her teens this patient was obese, and the menses were irregular until after the birth of the baby.

The first two remedies were ineffectual, but after a single dose of Lachesis 30c she had a normal menses without a headache for the first time for over twelve years, and did not report again for another thirteen months. She had occasional slight attacks thereafter, but these were not disabling, as they had previously been.

Not every case of migraine will clear up on a single remedy. I think of Mrs P., aged forty-two, a married woman with two children, who worked full time as a professional photographer. Her headaches were fortnightly – right-sided, preceded by a horizontal hemianopia, associated with repeated vomiting; the headache kept her in bed for forty-eight hours. Associated with the headache there was pain down the right arm from the elbow to the median three fingers; just before and during the attack there was a loss of colour vision. These additional symptoms suggested the possibility of a cerebral angioma, or an aneurysm of the circle of Willis. An X-ray of the skull was negative and an electro-encephalogram showed characteristics often associated with migraine.

She had had previous treatment with Sepia and Silica, without result. Repertorising the symptoms, Silica came out strongly, but so did Arsenicum and Nux Vomica. There was temporary improvement on Arsenicum, but – as Dr Borland used to point out – in the chronic case another remedy must be found to consolidate improvement from Arsenicum. Sulphur 30c was selected, but the patient's morale was upset by the sudden death of her mother, and it was four months before there was any response to what appeared to be well-indicated remedies. This was not the only time that I have seen a failure to react to a remedy after profound emotional disturbance. Subsequently there was a temporary response to Silica, but when the potency was raised to 200c there was a severe aggravation, and it was three months before any further improvement was noticed. Although this patient remained far from cured, the headaches were less severe and the intervals between the attacks were lengthening.

In treating very severe cases of migraine one must be prepared to persevere with treatment for a year or more, and to be prepared for relapses after a period of stress. Many homoeopaths will have found that once they have effected a cure of migraine, a whole series of patients are referred to them with periodic headaches. Not all of these are true migraine headaches and a number of them will be found to be tension headaches.

Tension Headaches

Mr R., aged forty-one, a plumber on the hospital staff, was passed on to me by a sceptical houseman, as he had failed to relieve him with ergotamine. He had flown fighter planes in World War II and his headaches dated from the time when he was piloting Meteors. The current RAF folklore about these aircraft was that the vibration was so terrific that the pilot became sterile. He had been in two crashes, but without personal injuries. His headaches occurred every three weeks, beginning in the morning with a tight band round the head, and accompanied by a bursting, throbbing sensation, worse on stooping. He had nausea but no vomiting with the headache. The scalp was very tender and his hat felt tight. The attack would last three days, during which he was unfit for work. He had a monthly dose of Belladonna 30c for six months. At the end of that time he had had four headaches, only one of which had lasted more than twelve hours.

He then had an accident in his car (Did this arouse subconscious memories of his plane crash?) and developed a phase of insomnia, recalling memories of his nightfighter days when he took amphetamine to keep awake. He responded to Coffea 6c each night for a month, and in the last six months had had only three headaches, in spite of worry about his wife's poor health.

Mrs M. M., aged forty-eight, with one child, menopause seven years previously, had severe headaches for thirteen years. Five days out of the week she awakened with a headache and could not bear light or noise or smells. Her teenage son developed schizophrenia but had made a good recovery, although since he was better he had become awkward and difficult at home, quarrelling with his father and upsetting his mother. She was a thin, dark, scrawny, very conscientious person, driving herself to do considerable voluntary work for the Red Cross. She improved on Sepia 200c, but her boy's wayward behaviour kept her on edge all the time. Ignatia 6c tided her over these recurrent crises, and occasional spaced doses of Sepia 200c reduced the frequency of the headaches to one every nine days. The headaches went off in an hour or two, so that she felt sufficiently confident to take up a job, which had the advantage of relieving her from the tense domestic atmosphere. She still had to endure the appalling scenes between father and son, but her physical reactions to these were much less severe, and considering the chronic stress under which she lived, I was surprised that I was able to help her as much as I did.

High Blood Pressure

Mr W. H., seventy-four, a widower, was referred to me because of headaches and giddiness. He was a tall, heavily-built man who had not yet retired from business, and still hunted with the Berkeley. Two years previously he had lost his wife after forty-five years of happy marriage. His headaches were occipital, and worse in the morning. He found it difficult to make decisions, could not tackle business problems, his memory had begun to fail, and he got hot and bothered. His doctor had kept him in bed for a fortnight, ordered him sedative tablets, and put him on a salt-free diet. However, he was not getting any better, and he had been giddy in bed and was troubled with tinnitus. His blood pressure was 200/125. He had a detached retina in one eye – the retinal vessels contracted in his good eye. I ordered China 30c, one dose. Three weeks later his headaches were better but his systolic pressure was still 190. I ordered him Sulphur 30c, and a fortnight later he returned saying he was altogether better, had followed the hunt once more, his tinnitus was less and he was walking five miles a day. In spite of (or because of) this his blood pressure was 220/130. A dose of Sulphur 200c was prescribed. Six weeks later he came to see me, feeling on top of the world. He had caught a cold watching a point-to-point on a very cold day, but apart from this all his symptoms were improved. His blood pressure was now 170/95. When I last saw him at the end of a year his systolic pressure was 165. He had had one more dose of Sulphur 200c in the interval. I learned later from his own doctor that he had married again and moved out of the country.

Growing Pains and Chilblains

In contrast to this septuagenarian here is the case of a teenager, worried about pains in her legs, with puffy ankles. She had chilblains in the cold. She was a typical Pulsatilla blonde and I ordered her a dose of the 1M potency. She wrote a month later to say that the only time her legs had ached was after a dance when she had done a great deal of jiving, and that her ankles did not now puff up when she got hot. A very severe winter followed, but in spite of this her legs remained much better. Throughout that winter she took a monthly dose of Pulsatilla 1M and was able to live an active life. She only once developed a small chilblain on one heel, whereas in previous winters she had been housebound with numerous severe chilblains.

Infected Toe

Mrs Y., a widow in her late fifties, had just taken up a post as housekeeper to a well-known citizen. Just before she started this work, in the process of trimming her toenails, she sliced a big toe and the wound became infected. She arrived in a carpet slipper and was limping around the mansion in great pain. Her doctor advised her to have the toenail removed, but she was reluctant to do this just as she was taking up a new post, as it would mean going into hospital. Hepar Sulph. 30c, four-hourly, relieved the splinter-like pains within a few hours and in a week the toe was healed. A minor event, but from the patient's point of view, nearly a major tragedy.

Acute Bursitis

Mrs M. D., aged fifty-two, a squat, dark-haired mother of a difficult teenage daughter, had never been well since her own mother had died fifteen years previously. Her older sister was in and out of the local psychiatric hospital for courses of ECT. Her neighbour's son was dying slowly of cancer. She felt that her husband and her daughter ganged up against her. Approaching the menopause, when she missed a period at the age of fifty-two, she accused her husband of being careless and spent several weeks convinced that she was pregnant. In these depressed moods she was accident-prone, and after a fall in the street, flat on her face, she turned up at Outpatients with a patellar bursitis. The skin over the knee was red and hot, and I suppose most casualty officers would have admitted her to hospital for incision and drainage. I knew, however, that this woman had a dread of hospitals. She had spent weeks of her life visiting her mother as well as the young neighbour dying of cancer; knowing her as I did, I was fairly certain that to admit her to hospital would precipitate a depressive illness. I therefore prescribed Belladonna 30c, four-hourly, and told her to rest at home. The week following she reported that she was walking normally, that there were no signs of inflammation and only a little fluid in the bursa.

Perennial Rhinitis
Mrs A., aged forty-five, was sent to me by her doctor for a rhinorr-hoea – a hay fever that persisted all the year round. She had seen an ENT specialist, had her sinuses X-rayed, and was ordered an anti-histamine. Her mother was an asthmatic. She herself had had nephritis eight years previously; soon after her discharge from hospital, her nose began to stream as soon as she woke, even while she was in bed. A cold draught would make her sneeze, and so would tobacco smoke. Her husband smoked all the time.

I prescribed Psorinum 30c, one dose. A month later she reported an aggravation on the seventh day, but since then had been free from rhinorrhoea and had taken no antihistamines for a whole month. This was the longest period she could remember without an attack. She was grateful for this relief, as she worked as a shorthand typist and her streaming nose had slowed her up considerably.

Enuresis
Michael, aged seven, was a boy of limited mentality who attended an occupation centre. He was enuretic and so smelly that the other children at the centre complained bitterly, and as a result he had been excluded. He was a gnome-like little boy with folded ears, undescended testes and a long foreskin. I ordered him Benzoic Acid 6c, three times a day, and three months later his mother reported that his diurnal enuresis had ceased, the urine was no longer offensive, and that he had returned to

the occupation centre, much to her relief, as she had younger children to care for. Previous investigation had demonstrated that one kidney was very small. This syndrome is often associated with folded helices of the ears, but in spite of the gross physical defect it was possible to effect considerable improvement in this boy's condition.

Psychogenic Bladder

Miss L., aged forty-four and unmarried, was sent to me by her doctor with a complex psychiatric history, as well as difficulty in micturition in any lavatory other than her home toilet. She had had a hysterectomy some years previously for fibroids and was taking imipramine for depression, a sedative for insomnia, and some fancy preparation for migraine. In the past she had been a soloist in an amateur operatic society, but could now no longer face the footlights, becoming grossly tremulous and unable to maintain breath control. Nothing abnormal was found on vaginal examination, but premenstrual tension was marked. She was liable to severe occipital headaches which extended forwards to either eye and were followed by vomiting of bile. Such a headache might last several days. As a child she had been liable to hysterical fits in which she lost the use of her left arm and voice. I prescribed Ambra Grisea 6c b.d. and she showed steady improvement in all respects, with satisfactory bladder function and no further need to take imipramine.

Osteoarthritis of the Hip

Mrs G., aged seventy, a general's widow, had suddenly gone lame after her husband's death four years before. She had had electric treatments, massage and short-wave diathermy without effect. X-rays showed advanced osteoarthritis of the right hip. She hobbled into my consulting room using two sticks. There was marked wasting of the thigh muscles and severe adductor spasm. There was severe pain referred to the knee. Movement of the right hip in all directions was severely limited.

Obviously one would not expect any medical treatment to alter the disorganisation and bony outgrowths round the hip joint, but it might still be possible to reduce the protective spasm of the muscles guarding the hip joint.

After taking the case, I prescribed Sulphur 200c, one dose, and Bellis Perennis 6c three times a day. She reported regularly by letter and came to see me a year later. She could move better and it was no longer agony to get into a car. She could climb into bed more easily; the thigh muscles were less wasted and there was an increase in range of movement of the right hip joint. Six months later she came to see me again, having in the interim had two doses of Sulphur 30c and two of Sulphur 200c. She was walking without sticks, could get into cars and buses without pain or difficulty, and was sleeping well. Indeed, she became so active that in the following year she developed a small varicose ulcer – she had many years ago suffered from phlebitis. A year later she was again active enough to become a victim of a coronary thrombosis, for which she was treated successfully. She still keeps in touch with me, has an occasional dose of Bryonia, but is able to walk without a stick.

On the face of it, this was a most unpromising case where physiotherapy had failed to give relief, and where very gross physical changes were present. Yet it was possible to render this patient from a practically housebound state to a relatively mobile condition. The change in her mental state was satisfactory too. From being a miserable, complaining, bitter old lady, she became a cheerful, dryly humorous philosopher who accepted her subsequent disabilities in an admirable way; one was able to appreciate the great qualities of this indomitable old lady that had been masked by the atrocious pain with which she had been plagued.

No case is hopeless. In spite of gross organic changes, even in elderly patients or in mentally-handicapped persons, there is a latent potential for response. By careful individualisation, it is possible with homoeopathic therapeutics to restore some capacity for worthwhile living to patients whose disabilities have presented an insoluble problem to orthodox medicine.

There is the story of the lady whose family doctor was trying to decide which specialist to send her to next. Like the classical case in the Gospels, she had suffered many things of many physicians, and was nothing bettered. As her doctor debated aloud about whom to send her next, the lady interrupted him – 'I want a doctor who will specialise in ME.' Of course the answer to the problem should have been a homoeopathic doctor, for that surely is our objective: we should be specialists in individuals.

Chapter 16

Some Plant Polychrests

Pulsatilla

As far back as seventy years ago, in the index of clinical cases collected for the Homoeopathic Society, Pulsatilla was prescribed for forty-nine different disorders. I have had a very successful result with the remedy in a patient with recurrent ulceration of the cornea, who had had no relief from a long series of consultant ophthalmologist prescriptions.

It has a long history. Dioscorides, an army surgeon at the time of Nero, refers to it; his *Materia Medica*, together with the writings of Hippocrates and Galen, formed the basis of European medicine for the next fourteen centuries, up to the time of the Renaissance. In 1771 Baron von Stork reintroduced Pulsatilla for chronic affections of the eyes.

British specimens of the plant are becoming rare and hard to find as more and more natural pasture is ploughed up. In the sixteenth century *Pulsatilla* formed purple patches on the Gog Magog hills in Cambridge-shire, and as late as 1930 a botanist wrote enthusiastically of a Cotswolds slope purple with the plant, but a distribution map printed in 1950 demonstrated to what extent it had disappeared from the countryside. Perhaps we can console ourselves that the British species has little medicinal power.

Some pharmacologists attribute the active principle to anemonine, whose chemical structure is closely connected with cantharidine; this is not relevant in practice as the whole plant extract is used in preparation of the remedy.

Margaret Tyler wrote that the classical description of the Pulsatilla patient is of a girl with sandy hair and blue eyes, pale face, easily moved to laughter or tears, with an affectionate, mild, timid, gentle, yielding disposition, and inclined to be fleshy. She says it is one of the easiest remedies to learn, but it is startling to note that there was not a single blonde among Dr Douglas McKellar's colour slides of patients treated with Pulsatilla (shown in a lecture given at the Faculty of Homoeopathy, London). They are all dark brunettes and some of them are quite slim. So Hahnemann's flaxen Saxons were not a true keynote.

Lycopodium

The next most frequently prescribed remedy in Dr English's investigation into the most frequently used remedies in a week of general practice in the 1970s was Lycopodium. Why did Hahnemann decide to prove this inert, waterproof yellowish powder, consisting of the sporules of club moss? It had been used to sprinkle over pills that stick easily together, and to dust over excoriated areas of human skin. It floats on liquid without being dissolved, and has no taste or smell. Microscopic examination shows that the particles are about one hundredth of an inch in diameter and shaped like a little nut. It takes at least two hours pounding in an agate mortar to fracture the envelope of these minute particles and release the oil globules that they contain.

Hahnemann was seventy-three when he published the first edition of *Chronic Diseases* in 1828, and the majority of the eight hundred and seventy symptoms attributed to Lycopodium are his own observations. Lycopodium was later re-proved in Germany in 1856 and 1859.

Lycopodium has been called the vegetable sulphur, for it was used to produce stage lighting in theatres. Sir George Porter gave a beautiful demonstration at the Royal Institution in his televised lecture on the natural history of a sunbeam, by blowing Lycopodium powder through the flame of a Bunsen burner. Dr Sankaran of Bombay comments that Lycopodium symptoms may also come in a flash. They can be sudden and intense, as for example sudden hunger or sexual excitement. But the satisfaction or satiety is also very quick and sudden. He considers that its aluminium content may explain many of these features.

Dr Tyler used to say that to become a rapid and correct prescriber there are a dozen remedies that one needs to make friends with, so as to be able to recognise them with a minimum of glances and questioning, and that Lycopodium is one of them. Clarke writes that there will be some symptoms which are peculiarly characteristic of the remedy – the keynotes.

Prescribing on keynotes alone is an absurdity, he says, but the right use of keynotes is an immense saving of labour. He lists no less than eleven keynotes, including the aggravation from 4–8 p.m., the right-to-left progression, the improvement from uncovering, which is the opposite to Silica. The Lycopodium patient is better from warm food and drinks, and worse from cold food. Dr David Wilson has called attention to the fan-like motion of the alae nasi in disorders of children. The movements are usually rapid, never slow, and are not synchronous with the respiration.

Clarke warns about the frequency of aggravations after a high potency of Lycopodium, and indeed has discouraged some prescribers from using this valuable remedy. Hahnemann had foreseen this, and recommended Pulsatilla to counteract the feverish aggravations, and Causticum for the ill-humour – taking things in the wrong way, the mistrust and the reproaches. Coffea, Hahnemann claimed, extinguishes the action of Lycopodium. It is the experience of many homoeopaths that repeated doses of Lycopodium are much less effective than in the first instance.

Thuja
Hahnemann gives no reason as to why he selected *Thuja occidentalis* or *Arbor vitae* for proving in the fifth volume of his *Materia Medica*. He cited no Old School authorities and it does not seem to have been employed in official medicine. Hugh Johnson, in his splendid book on trees, asserts that *Thuja* was the first American tree to be grown in . Europe, and that there was a record of one in Paris in 1553. Eric Newby in *The World Atlas of Exploration* records how Cartier's expedition of 1542 was spent with their ships frozen deep in the ice of the St Lawrence River in Canada from November to mid-April. The crew suffered intensely from scurvy, but eventually the scurvy was cured with the juice of a tree, *Thuja occidentalis*. Some of the sailors even alleged that it cured the syphilis from which they had been suffering for years. The tree of life, *Arbor vitae*, indeed. No wonder Cartier brought such a treasure home to France. In those days gonorrhoea and syphilis were regarded as due to the same infecting agent, and it may well have been that the French sailors were suffering from a chronic gonoccocal infection.

Dr Dudgeon, sometime Editor of the *British Journal of Homoeopathy*, relates the following experience. 'Last July, when taking a walk, I happened to pass a thuja tree laden with green cones. I plucked one, chewed it a little and thought no more about it. That same evening I observed a very disagreeable scalding on making water, which continued all next day, and I was horrified to observe on undressing that my shirt was spotted all over in a manner extremely repugnant to one's notions of respectability. I found a considerable bleeding discharge from the urethra, which was evidently swollen and inflamed, as the stream of urine was small and split and the burning had increased. I had quite forgotten the circumstance of having chewed the thuja cone the previous day, and could not imagine what could have produced in a decent paterfamilias such a very incongruous complaint. The following day the discharge had become yellow but the other symptoms remained as before. I now remembered chewing the cone and regarded the malady with more composure. The discharge still continued, though in a diminished degree, until the sixth day, and on the seventh day I was again quite well.' This is, as Dr Dudgeon commented, a picture of acute gonorrhoea. Borland describes the Thuja child as under average height, with a tendency to subnormality and easily upset by onions and tea. In his experience, bad teeth due to defects in the enamel were a common feature.

Ignatia

Ignatia is prepared from the seeds of *Strychnos ignatia*, a close relative of *Strychnos nux vomica*, but the *Ignatia* is a much more elegant tree than *Nux vomica*, with long, smooth branches, in contrast with the short, crooked, knotted branches of *Nux vomica*. The *Nux vomica* flowers are nothing out of the ordinary, but the *Ignatia* inflorescence is strikingly beautiful; an umbel of nine to ten white flowers, each a tube some nine inches long, ending in a white, five-pointed star enclosing the five long stamens and the thread-like stele. The fruit is a large berry as big as a medium-size pear, with a thick, woody coat containing numerous hard seeds. Hahnemann advises keeping the mortar standing in very hot water in order to triturate these hard seeds through the first three potencies. It was a Jesuit monk who first brought the seeds from the Philippine Islands to the notice of Portuguese merchants. He called them St Ignatius's beans in honour of the founder of the Jesuits, Ignatius Loyola. The natives wore the seeds as amulets for the prevention or cure of a variety of diseases. The seeds reached Holland at the end of the seventeenth century.

Ignatia was one of the twenty-five remedies whose provings Hahnemann first published in 1805 in his *Fragmenta Medica*. Ignatia had one hundred and seventy-six 'fragments' or symptoms. But he had already referred to Ignatius's Bean in an essay in Hufeland's *Journal* nine years earlier, containing suggestions for ascertaining the curative powers of drugs, so that in the third edition of his *Materia Medica* thirty-seven years later he had had plenty of time to identify the type of person most susceptible to Ignatia.

Unlike Nux Vomica, he said that Ignatia is not suitable for persons in whom anger, eagerness or violence is preponderant. But it is suitable for those who are subject to rapid alternations of gaiety and disposition to weep. They have no tendency to break out violently or to revenge themselves, but keep their annoyance to themselves. Hahnemann recommended that Ignatia should be taken in the morning, because if given shortly before bed-time it causes too much restlessness. The patients are over-sensitive to pain but, nevertheless, bear their pain patiently, at the worst with quiet weeping. But in contrast to Pulsatilla the characteristic Ignatia reaction to grief is sighing rather than weeping. The Ignatia patient cannot stand smoking or tobacco smoke, and the Ignatia child is liable to prolapse of the rectum. Dr Borland regretted the tendency in some textbooks to regard Ignatia as corresponding to a hysterical female. He saw it as indicated for the highly-strung, sensitive, bright, precocious child who was doing well at school, but who was being pushed too hard by ambitious parents or teachers.

Stramonium
The thorn-apple, *Datura stramonium*, is a herb which in Britain occurs casually on rubbish and manure heaps. Originally it came from the countries round the Caspian Sea. From Constantinople the herbalist Gerard received some seeds at the end of the sixteenth century, and cultivated the plant. Meanwhile, this alien plant had also reached Italy and from there was introduced into Germany, and is now widely distributed over Europe. The Viennese physician Storck introduced it into medicine in the middle of the eighteenth century, although the Chinese had used Stramonium as a prophylactic against rabies for many years; in classical times it was used in oracles and in medieval times by wizards.

Stramonium too, was one of the first twenty-five remedies proved by Hahnemann and published in his *Fragmenta* in 1805. In his introduction to the remedy in the *Materia Medica*, first published twenty years later, he claims, 'I speak from experience of its incomparable curative action in mental maladies and convulsive ailments', and comments on the absence of pain in the provings.

In some forms of scarlet fever Stramonium may be better than Belladonna, but its main indications are the hallucinations and delirium of acute mania and delirium tremens. Kent says that Stramonium is like an earthquake in its violence, and Borland said that immediately you get terrors in the symptomatology you begin to think of Stramonium. Tyler reported a case of threatened acute mastoiditis which made no improvement on Hepar Sulph., but two days later the patient was very agitated, clasping and unclasping her hands, moving her feet and swaying her body. Diplomatic questioning revealed that she felt deserted and forlorn, and that she had a fear of rushing water. Within twenty-four hours of a prescription of Stramonium 1M the girl's distressing symptoms had disappeared and the condition of the ear greatly improved. In 1971 the *British Medical Journal* contained a short report on the misuse of herbal cigarettes containing stramonium. An art student of twenty-five and a sixteen-year-old girl were both admitted to hospital with histories of collapse and bizarre behaviour after eating a couple of herbal cigarettes.

Aethusa

Aethusa or fool's parsley, or dog-parsley in Somerset, is a common weed in town gardens. It was confused with hemlock, *Conium*, and a Dr Harvey of St Thomas' Hospital, London complained that in a series of experiments large doses of the juice were entirely inoperative. But later researches by a Dr Power demonstrated the presence of a very small quantity of a volatile poisonous principle identical with hemlock.

The homoeopathic tincture is made from the whole fresh plant. As far back as 1796, Hahnemann found himself distracted and incapable of reading any more because of much mental work coming upon him in rapid succession, and he took a grain of a good extract of *Aethusa* that he had prepared himself. The effect was an uncommon disposition for mental labour which lasted for several hours. Clarke reports on an undergraduate preparing for an examination who had been compelled to give up his studies because of his inability to think or fix his attention. Given this remedy he was able to resume work and passed a brilliant examination. Dr Margaret Tyler comments that this condition of working to the limits for an examination, when it is useless to attempt any further study, and when the student may even refuse to go into the examination room, is a condition of stalemate and must not be confused with the Argentum Nitricum state, which is examination nerves – a condition of acute anxiety and apprehension, even ending in diarrhoea.

A French physician spoke very highly of its value in intolerance of milk in children, and this was confirmed by the American Dr Guernsey. The child vomits milk in large curds, is weak and exhausted after vomiting, and falls asleep only to wake up hungry, to eat and vomit again. Nash describes the very characteristic facies of these children; a sunken face with a marked linear crease, the upper lip is pearly-white. Kent goes even further and defines it as a Hippocratic face.

Capsicum

It is difficult to discover how the next remedy reached Europe. *Capsicum*, the red pepper or chilli, is a cultivated South American plant which is reported to have reached Hungary in 1585. It is very rich in vitamin C. Hahnemann called it Spanish pepper and reported his first provings in his *Fragmenta*. He said that diseases curable by Capsicum are rarely met with in persons of tense fibre. One of his symptoms was a swelling on the bone behind the ear, painful to the touch. The American Allen followed this up, and Capsicum has proved valuable in threatened mastoid; Hughes confirmed this in a personal case where he had expected to resort to surgery, but where the patient made a complete recovery with preservation of hearing. Another of Hahnemann's symptoms, the coughing spells and offensive breath from the lung, led to the successful prescription of Capsicum in the case of an abscess of the lung. It was Clarke who drew attention to the homesickness, with red cheeks and sleeplessness. He cured an Australian student who had come to London and was quite incapacitated with homesickness. It has proved valuable in the children's ward where recently admitted children are found inconsolable. The children are fat, flabby and red-faced, but their red noses are often cold. They are thirsty, but drinking makes them shiver. Dr Borland said that he had never seen a neat Capsicum child. He found them lazy, somewhat obstinate, very definitely clumsy, rather dull and slow to learn, with a poor memory.

Chamomilla

In the British Isles there are three native species of camomile, including the lawn camomile. But none of them is Hahnemann's Chamomilla, which is a mayweed, *Matricaria chamomilla*. In contrast to the common scentless mayweed, our *Chamomilla* is not frequently found. It is a sweetly aromatic plant; its close relative, the pineapple weed or rayless mayweed, is even more aromatic. Dioscorides included camomile in his *Materia Medica*, and Culpeper recommended it in his *Complete Herbal and Physician* to remedy such infirmities as a careless midwife has caused. In Hahnemann's time the physicians called it a domestic remedy; rather than prescribe vulgar folk remedies they ordered *Anthemis nobilis*, which possesses different properties and actions. Hughes, who was no botanist, considered there was no difference between them.

Hahnemann reported in 1796 on the results when he gave a pregnant woman an overdose of the volatile oil of camomile. His first proving was printed nine years later in the *Fragmenta* and an expanded proving was published in his *Materia Medica*. He quoted only three Old School authorities. Apart from his pupil Stapf, who observed the symptoms in a girl of nineteen who had drunk some cupfuls of strong camomile tea, all the symptoms were Hahnemann's own observations.

He attached great importance to his experience that it was not suitable for persons who bear pain patiently and calmly. Chamomilla was re-proved by the Vienna Provers Union and the Americans expanded the use of the remedy. Dr Durham pointed out that the colic was worse from warmth, in contrast to the colic which is relieved by warmth; Dr Guernsey mentioned the spiteful, sudden, uncivil irascibility. The same doctor pointed out that the teething infant will not be soothed unless it is carried about. Clarke says that the Chamomilla patient cannot be civil to the doctor; unlike Aconite and Arsenicum, the restless Chamomilla patient would rather die than so suffer. It has been found useful in the withdrawal stage of heroin addicts. Chamomilla will always stop the vomiting from morphine after the crude effects of the drug have passed away. Dr Borland pointed out the similarity of symptoms whether it was Arsenicum or Chamomilla: the myoclonic seizure, the restlessness, the intense pains. The Chamomilla child is in a frenzy of rage; it resents the pain, it is perfectly furious that you have not cleared it off at once. You do your best for the Chamomilla child but it is liable to hit you. You start jogging a Chamomilla child and it will probably stop its yelling and begin to crow. You stop and it wants you to go on, and if you do not it will pull your hair.

Abrotanum
The next two remedies are both wormwoods. There are an enormous number of wormwoods botanically, something like four hundred, but the first to be described is *Artemisia abrotanum*, known as lad's love or lady's love, and it was another plant described by Dioscorides and listed by Culpeper. The English botanists found it in Russia in the seventeenth century. It was in great demand in London in the 1770s as it could tolerate the smoke, unlike many garden plants. When the leaf is held up against the light, the oil glands show up as transparent dots. Clarke emphasises its wasting, particularly of the legs, in spite of the ravenous appetite. The face is pale, wrinkled, old-looking and feels cold. He cured a woman of indigestion associated with vomiting large quantities of offensive fluid. Was it a case of pyloric obstruction? Nash speaks of marasmus of children whose skin hangs in loose folds. Borland indentified the cause of the wasting as congenital pyloric stenosis. It is always a cross and peevish baby because it is starving. Older children, he says, are also very hungry and suffer from diarrhoea alternating with rheumatism. Kent says the diarrhoea is a great relief and that is when the Abrotanum patients are at their best. Margaret Tyler endorses these points and indicates that unlike Aethusa, the hungry Abrotanum child craves bread and milk. It is an extremely cross, ill-natured child with a cruel, sadistic streak in its make-up.

Cina

The other Artemisia is *Artemisia cina* (commonly referred to as Cina in the homoeopathic materia medica). This variety of wormwood grows on the steppes, east of the Aral Sea in Russian Central Asia. The chief characteristic of this steppe is the low growth of the plants belonging to it, these being separated by wide stretches of bare soil and by the predominance of the uniform, grey foliage. In the autumn, from among the dismembered plants battered by the strong, dry east winds, there springs up a fresh vegetation of *Artemisia* which can cover whole tracts with pure masses of wormwood. The local tribesmen collect the plant and market it. Hippocrates recommended it as a vermifuge, as well as for the seeds, which contain santonin and were specially collected. The trouble is that the plant must ripen seeds, but as it matures, the wind scatters a good part of it, where it is lost. As the collectors dare not touch it by hand for fear of losing the seed, they take two hand-baskets and, walking along the steppes, sweep the baskets one from right to left, and the other from left to right as if they were mowing. Santonin, the active principle, is insoluble in water. Hahnemann recommended macerating the buds in alcohol, but later pharmacists recommended triturating the first three potencies.

Hahnemann listed only forty-eight symptoms in the first edition of the *Materia Medica*, but the third edition has three hundred and one, and the last symptom is, 'Cannot be quieted by any persuasion'; it is this obstinacy, obstinate as a mule, that for Borland distinguishes Cina from Chamomilla. Hughes prefers crude doses of santonin as a vermifuge, but quotes a French doctor for its value in whooping cough. Cina is much more than a mere worm medicine. It has cured typhoid. Special features are the tense, circumscribed redness of the cheeks, the violent rubbing of the nose, the excessive hunger even after a full meal. If you see a yawning child picking its nose, always explore the possibility of its being a Cina patient. Margaret Tyler says that the Cina child cannot be punished, because it goes into a convulsion.

Chapter 17

Homoeopathy and Research

The *Oxford Dictionary* defines 'empiric' as 'based on observation and experiment, not on theory' – whence empiricist, a person relying solely on experiment – a quack! By the beginning of the 18th century, the age of authoritarian dogma was coming to an end; there was a wariness about too many hypotheses and an interest and respect for the tangible and visible.

Sir Harold Himworth, when Secretary of the Medical Research Council, stated, 'There are only two kinds of scientific activity: investigations aimed at understanding naturally-occurring phenomena – research; and investigations into the application of knowledge gained and human needs – development.' Homoeopathic medicine fulfils both these requirements. It is based on experimental pharmacology – the provings; and on clinical experience – the application of the knowledge gained by the provings.

Here homoeopaths are in the best of company. Jenner's observations on vaccination were the foundations of immunology, and it was Fleming's observation that led to the discovery of antibiotics, although the accumulation of observations by themselves does not necessarily lead to progress. The pedantic mind considers it unethical to generalise beyond the evidence. Yet that is what all great hypotheses do. The discovery itself is of necessity always intuitive, if it is really new. Hahnemann's observations on his personal experiments with cinchona bark led him to the great generalisation of *similia similibus curentur*. Empiricists or rationalists? Surely we need a combination of both.

It has been claimed that the basic texture of research consists of dreams into which the threads of reasoning, measurement and calculation are woven. Hahnemann also wrote, 'We know life only by its symptoms.' What better confirmation of his dictum in the *Organon* that 'only the changes in health of body and mind which can be perceived externally by means of the senses' can guide us in the selection of the remedy?

After twenty years study of vital processes, Szent-Györgyi, the discoverer of Vitamin C, pointed out, 'There is a basic difference between physics and biology. Physics is the science of probabilities. If a process goes 999 times one way and only once the other way, the physicist will not hesitate to accept the first. Biology is the science of the improbable, and it is a principle that the body works only with reactions which are statistically improbable. If metabolism were built on a series of probable and thermodynamically spontaneous reactions, then we would burn up and the machine would run down as a watch does if deprived of its regulators. The reactions are kept in hand by being statistically improbable, and made possible by specific tricks which may then be used for regulation. Reactions are possible in living organisms which seem impossible, or at least improbable, to the physicist.'

Hahnemann's pharmacological experiments began in 1805. These were the first organised provings, but before 1790, when he translated Cullen's *Materia Medica*, he had already published thirty-one books and articles, and was recognised as one of the leading scientists of his day. He had met and discussed with Lavoisier. He had made careful experiments on crystallisation. He had investigated the fermentation of wine in a series of elaborate experiments involving succussion, as he realised the importance of repeated contact. He had researched into the adulteration of drugs and had devised tests that were sensitive enough to detect contamination to a degree of one part in 30,000. As one contemporary reviewer pointed out, 'Accuracy prevails everywhere – melting-points, specific gravities, solubilities in water and alcohol.' He invented new apparatus and devised new techniques for reducing all sorts of substances to powder.

His pharmacological experiments were confirmed by independent observers, who had hoped to refute his findings. Particularly of note were the re-provings of Jörg in 1825 and the Vienna Society of Physicians. It was soon recognised that all the symptoms a remedy can produce are not observable in one person only, and that it was necessary to test it on many subjects. Hahnemann did not recognise hereditary maladies, although Dudgeon, the Victorian homoeopath, considered that congenital faulty constitutions must be regarded as one great source of chronic disease.

Recent research has shown that individuals vary in the rate at which they metabolise drugs. For example, isoniazid and sulphadimidine are inactivated by enzymes which acetylate these drugs in the liver. Individuals can be classified as slow or rapid inactivators. The slow inactivators can be expected to produce more side effects – that is, proving richer in symptoms. It has been suggested that the victims of asbestosis are those members of the population who have inherited a tendency to produce abnormal quantities of antiglobulin and antinuclear factors, and so are predisposed to lung changes.

Chronic disease was a challenge to Hahnemann. To try to find the solution he proved another forty-seven drugs between 1816 and 1828. These included such invaluable remedies as Calcarea Carb., Causticum, Graphites, Kali Carb., Lycopodium, Natrum Mur., Phosphorus, Sepia and Silica. Without these experiments we should be seriously handi-capped today. We may not find his theories of chronic disease acceptable now, but his clinical observations on the conduct of the treatment of these illnesses are still relevant. Modern investigations give support to his notes on aggravations and suppressions and the importance of time-dependent changes in symptoms.

Recent progress in immunology has shown the complicated relation-ship of the two main defence systems of the body – the immunoglobulins in the plasma and the sensitised lymphocyte cells.

Dr Turk has shown how in chronic infections such as leprosy and syphilis, at different stages of the illness, one or other of these two different defence mechanisms either come into action or fail, so that patients do not stay at the same point. At one extreme the cells are the chief defenders, at the other end of the scale the plasma globulins take up the struggle.

Treatment will upset the balance, so that the roles of the defence mechanisms are reversed and symptoms characteristic of the first stages of the illness recur, particularly with regard to skin eruptions. It is encouraging to have a scientific explanation of the observations familiar to us homoeopaths for nearly two centuries. Of course there are still many unsolved problems in homoeopathic medicine, as there are in biology. There are still unknown reactions which in scientific slang are labelled 'blackbox' reactions, which researchers hope to clarify later.

One promising line of enquiry is the research into the water of crystallisation. It has been shown that the water molecules arrange themselves in ever more complicated polyhedra around the chemical in the crystal, and the evidence suggests that this holds good for substances in solution. What is fascinating is that around the larger organic molecules as many as 136 molecules of water are built up in a complicated lattice encircling the guest molecule. These hydrates are stable up to 40°C and tend to be unique in structure and interaction – in other words, specific.

Another interesting item in the research on the structure of solutions is that air also participates, to some extent, in stabilising the lattice structures by being trapped within some of the open cages. What price succussion now?

It is now possible to consider recent findings in pharmacological research and to try and relate these results with the basic provings, as recorded by Hahnemann's team, and finally to see what bearing these results have on the conduct of modern provings.

There are a number of examples of involuntary provings in the literature. The *British Medical Journal* published a paper which homoeopathic physicians might classify as a series of involuntary provings of the muscle relaxant suxamethonium. One of the most dramatic symptoms after this drug is given is the cessation of respiration. Now suxamethonium is used as a relaxant by anaesthetists, but it is disconcerting to both anaesthetist and surgeon when a patient undergoing a straightforward operation for varicose veins, squint, tonsillectomy or dilatation and curettage, stops breathing and needs what is euphemistically called controlled ventilation, for periods ranging from an hour or more before normal respiration is resumed. In most people, suxamethonium is destroyed rapidly by the enzyme pseudocholinesterase. It has been found, however, that some people possess an atypical form of the enzyme which has only a slight effect on the breakdown of suxamethonium. In these persons the effect of the relaxant will be dangerously prolonged. Further investigation has shown that the possession of this abnormal enzyme is an inherited defect, which an anaesthetist is likely to meet about once in every thousand cases in the anaesthetic room.

In the paper referred to above, seven examples of this sensitivity to suxamethonium were encountered in nine months. Using a recently-developed test it was shown that twenty-two relatives, parents, siblings, or children of six of these cases were also sensitive to suxamethonium. The reagents in this test are employed in the equivalent of the fifth decimal potency.

The implication for the research worker is that in the case of suxamethonium only one out of a thousand possible provers would be likely to show a full range of symptoms – only one in a thousand patients would show indications for this remedy if prescribed homoeopathically. If a sensitive prover of one sex were found, it would be worth persuading a relative of the opposite sex to prove the remedy as well, to get a full range of its potential symptomatology. If a good therapeutic result occurred in one patient, it would be reasonable to expect that other members of the family might also respond to the same remedy.

To alter our range, we can turn to more mundane matters and note the effect of beetroot on certain individuals. Three Glasgow doctors investigated the reasons why some people excrete pink urine after eating beetroot. Only some people 'prove' beetroot in this way – one person in every seven. At first it was thought to be a hereditary phenomenon, but further tests threw doubt on this. The doctors showed that excretion of betacyanin, the red-violet pigment, was not an allergic symptom but related to iron deficiency and iron-deficient anaemic subjects. The theoretical significance of this is that certain symptoms will not be observed in apparently perfectly healthy people.

Another example, in the field of pharmacogenetics – the study of genetically-determined variations that are revealed by the effect of drugs – was accidentally discovered in the course of treatment. In 1952 a Japanese ear, nose and throat surgeon, Takahara, was cleaning out the maxillary sinus of a patient with hydrogen peroxide when he noticed that no frothing occurred on the raw surface, and that the free blood adjacent to it turned black. He suspected that there might be a deficiency in the patient's blood of the enzyme catalase, which breaks down peroxide into water and oxygen. When his patient's blood was tested, it was found to be totally deficient in this enzyme. Further investigation has discovered thirty-eight individuals in seventeen families with a similar deficiency. These patients have a predisposition to dental sepsis and ulceration of the gums, and eventually lose all their teeth.

Again, orthodox physicians treating tuberculosis with isoniazid soon discovered that there were two kinds of patients; either they were good excretors of the drug or poor excretors. It was shown that the rate of excretion depended on an inherited factor. The slow excretors were eight times more likely to develop polyneuritis after isoniazid than the good excretors. An observation comparing patients from different countries showed that there was little difference between Caucasians, Africans and Madras Indians, who were all poor excretors, whereas Japanese and Eskimos were nearly all good excretors and therefore very unlikely to develop polyneuritis. In other words, to 'prove' isoniazid on Japanese subjects would result in a very imperfect picture.

The deficiency of a vitamin can modify or intensify the effects of a drug. In Nigeria, paediatricians encountered a problem when prescribing a vitamin or its analogue, for example vitamin K, to newborn babies; this was intended to act in the prevention of haemorrhagic disease in the neonate. It was observed that some of these babies, instead of developing bleeding, developed jaundice, and further that some of these jaundiced babies had a deficiency of the enzyme glucose-6 phosphate dehydrogenase (G-6 P.D.). This deficiency of G-6 P.D. is fairly frequently found in Africans, and indeed about one in seven are affected. It is sex-linked. The condition was first discovered during the course of anti-malarial therapy and was termed primaquine sensitivity; these subjects develop toxic symptoms not only after primaquine but also after phenacetin, sulphanilamide, naphthalene and several other drugs. As the anomaly is sex-linked, one should expect different results from using men and women provers where this enzyme deficiency is prevalent.

For a long time Jamaicans have used a periwinkle extract in the domestic treatment of diabetes; this is *Vinca rosea*, the source of the alkaloid vinblastine which has produced remarkable remissions in lymphadenoma. When Canadian and American investigators analysed periwinkle extracts they failed to find an oral hypoglycaemic action. Perhaps their testers were Caucasians and not enzyme-deficient like the Jamaicans.

Another example of the effect of a deficiency of this particular enzyme is the haemolytic anaemia that is a consequence of a diet of broad beans. This illness, known in the textbooks as favism, occurs in natives of Calabria, the Balkans and North Africa. A similar mechanism may be at work in lathyrism, due to eating the pea *Lathyrus sativus*. *Vinca* and *Lathyrus* are very closely associated botanical genera. In Clarke's *Dictionary*, cases of lathyrism were collected from Italy and Algiers, the same population liable to favism. Clarke comments that men are more sensitive to lathyrus poisoning than women. I have never been impressed with the results of Lathyrus in polio-like illnesses in Britain. It may be that few Caucasians are sensitive to it. However, this particular enzyme deficiency has been observed in Caucasians as well as Africans. It has been observed that while the effects of drugs like vitamin K in Africans are only slight, in deficient Caucasians they can be severe. This difference in effects is believed to be genetic. The corollary follows that the results of proving certain drugs on Caucasians and Africans might differ considerably. It may be said that this is only a theoretical consideration; but Hering's organisation of provings in the United States were carried out at a time before the American Civil War, when negro provers were unlikely to have been included. Did Hahnemann use some of Hering's provings in his lists for Arsenicum, Natrum Carb., Phosphoric Acid and Silica?

As Hughes points out, the number of remedies in whose proving Hering has taken a more or less principal part is only less than that which we owe to Hahnemann. Quite apart from his heroic personal provings of Lachesis, we are indebted to Hering for Apis, Glonoine, Benzoic Acid,

Aloes, Allium Cepa, Natrum Sulph., Fluoric Acid, Oxalic Acid, Kalmia, Podophyllum, Eupatorium and Sanguinaria.

That this particular enzyme deficiency is not without significance in other parts of the world is demonstrated by a paper from Thailand, where the chief of the blood bank in Bangkok showed that G-6 P.D. deficiency may rise to 17.8% of the population in the foothills, whereas in the mountains it varied from only 0–3%. These findings were important, as it could be shown that people with this enzyme defect were resistant to malaria. What drugs would these subjects be resistant to as well as to the malarial parasite?

Dr Fraser Roberts, author of *An Introduction to Medical Genetics*, considers it likely that many more genetically-determined drug sensitivities will be discovered in the near future. It may well be that our most sensitive provers to particular remedies react as a function of their particular genetic constitution. If this is so, it would not be unreasonable to expect that such provers would react similarly to different substances used in provings, and that there would be an overlap in the symptomatology produced by these different substances.

Appendix

Publications

Papers on Homoeopathy

1928

The Homoeopathy of Lactation. *Bristol Homoeopathic Journal*, **18**, 12–24.

The Relation of Homoeopathy to Modern Conceptions of the Psychoses (the first Leopold Salzer Prize Essay). *British Homoeopathic Journal*, **18**, 140–68: 227–61.

The Rubrics of the Duodenal Syndrome. *British Homoeopathic Journal*, **18**, 342–5.

1929

The Homoeopathic Treatment of Asthma. *British Homoeopathic Journal*, **19**, 311–14.

1930

Generals. *British Homoeopathic Journal*, **20**, 110–38.

1931

The Foresight of Hahnemann. *Homoeopathic World*, **66**, 275–90.

The Next Prescription. *British Homoeopathic Journal*, **21**, 133–44.

On Migraine, its Aetiology and Treatment. *Medical Press and Circular*, **109**, 12–13.

On the Importance of Constitution as Influencing Treatment. *Medical Press and Circular*, **109**, 366.

Osteoarthritis and Rheumatoid Arthritis. *Medical Press and Circular*, **110**, 78.

1932

Menopausal Types and their Homoeopathic Treatment. *Medical Press and Circular*, **110**, 140–1.

The Contribution of Hahnemann to Modern Medicine. *Medical Press and Circular*, **110**, 175.

Right and Left Remedies; is there a Biological Explanation? *Actes du Congrès International d'Homéopathie.* Paris, 290–5.

1933

The Contribution to Medicine made by Samuel Hahnemann. *Janus*, **88**, 247–56.

El Peligro de las Prescripsiones basadas en los tipicos constituccionales. *El Sol de Meissen*, 329–31.

British Homoeopathy during the Last Hundred Years (with Sir John Weir). *British Homoeopathic Journal*, **23**, 3–8.

The Homoeopathic Remedy as the Detector of Latent Septic Foci. *British Homoeopathic Journal*, **23**, 368–73.

1934

Reflexions d'un Uniciste. *Propagateur d'Homeopathie*, 551–6.

1935

Scientific Provings versus Clinical Empiricism. *British Homoeopathic Journal*, **25**, 110–29.

English Provings of Naja. *Transactions International Homoeopathic Congress*. Budapest.

1936

Levels of Drug Action. *British Homoeopathic Journal*, **26**, 19–32.

The Evolution of the Lycopodium Drug Picture. *British Homoeopathic Journal*, **26**, 416–33.

1937

The Pathology of the Snake Venoms. *British Homoeopathic Journal*, **27**, 211–16.

1938

Silica, a Study in Mineral Balance. *British Homoeopathic Journal*, **28**, 130–42.

Tarentula Hispanica. *British Homoeopathic Journal*, **28**, 249–50.

1939

The Present-day Confirmation of the Homoeopathic Approach. *British Homoeopathic Journal*, **29**, 1–15.

Constitution and Chronic Disease. *British Homoeopathic Journal*, **29**, 224–41.

1941

The Homoeopathic Treatment of Allergic Conditions. *British Homoeopathic Journal*, **31**, 225–34.

1945

Proposed Group of Homoeopathy. Council Meeting B.M.A. *British Medical Journal Supplement*, 23 June, 124.

1946

Learning and Teaching Homoeopathy. *British Homoeopathic Journal*, **36**, 154–60.

1948

Homoeopathy. *Chambers' Encyclopaedia*.

1949

Homoeopathy and the Psychosomatic Approach. *British Homoeopathic Journal*, **39**, 127–37.

1951

The General Adaptation Theory of Selye and its Relation to Homoeopathic Theory. *Report of International Homoeopathic Congress*. Lausanne.

Basic Concepts of Homoeopathy. *Surgo, Glasgow University Medical Journal*, 41–4.

Publications

1952

The Place of Homoeopathy in Psychiatry. *British Homoeopathic Journal*, **43**, 27–33.

Homoeopathy in Psychiatry. *Proceedings of the International Homoeopathic Congress*. The Hague.

1954

Lecture delivered to the Osler Society, Oriel College, Oxford. *British Homoeopathic Journal*, **44**, 69–75.

Presidential Address, British Homoeopathic Congress, Bristol. *British Homoeopathic Journal*, **44**, 166–74.

1955

Oration: Bicentenary of Hahnemann. *British Homoeopathic Journal*, **45**, 7–13.

1956

Presidential Address. *British Homoeopathic Journal*, **45**, 48–55.

1957

Migraine. *British Homoeopathic Journal*, **46**, 94–5.

1958

Some Observations on the Treatment of Neuroses in Childhood. *British Homoeopathic Journal*, **47**, 4–13.

Valedictory Address. *British Homoeopathic Journal*, **47**, 313–15.

1959

Obituary: David Morgan Hughes. *British Homoeopathic Journal*, **48**, 83.

Salzburg Impressions. *British Homoeopathic Journal*, **48**, 153–4.

Homoeopathy and Scientific Standards. *Der wissenschaftliche Rahmen der Homöopathie*, Stuttgart, and *British Homoeopathic Journal*, **48**, 153–4.

1960

Sir John Weir's Anniversary. *British Homoeopathic Journal*, **49**, 150–1.

1961

The Life and Times of Dr Quin. *British Homoeopathic Journal*, **50**, 73–82.

Obituary: Dr. Borland. *British Homoeopathic Journal*, **50**, 134.

Congress Impressions (report on British Homoeopathic Congress, London 1961). *British Homoeopathic Journal*, **50**, 282–3.

1962

Wider Issues. *British Homoeopathic Journal*, **51**, 51–4.

Genes, Drugs, and Sensitivity. *British Homoeopathic Journal*, **51**, 83.

1963

Some Clinical Observations. *British Homoeopathic Journal*, **52**, 249–55.

The Improbability of Life (annotation). *British Homoeopathic Journal*, **52**, 275.

1964

Provers. *British Homoeopathic Journal*, **53**, 161–9.

1966

The Chronic Outpatient. *British Homoeopathic Journal*, **55**, 7–10.

My Introduction to Homoeopathy. *British Homoeopathic Journal*, **55**, 210–15.

1967

The Scope of Homoeopathy. *British Homoeopathic Journal*, **56**, 67–74.

Translation of Charette's 'My Introduction to Homoeopathy'. *British Homoeopathic Journal*, **56**, 80–5.

1968

The Role of Homoeopathic Medicine in the National Health Service. *Lancet*, **1**, 913–14.

Treatment of Hypertension in Elderly Subjects. *British Homoeopathic Journal*, **57**, 210–15.

1970

Richard Hughes Memorial Lecture. *British Homoeopathic Journal*, **59**, 179–93.

1971

Empiricism. *British Homoeopathic Journal*, **60**, 26–8.

Book Review (Hormones and the Immune Response). *British Homoeopathic Journal*, **60**, 111–12.

Homoeopathy. *Nursing Mirror*, **86**, 36–7.

Psychiatric Disorders of Old Age. *British Homoeopathic Journal*, **60**, 185–91.

Obituary: Sir John Weir. *British Homoeopathic Journal*, **60**, 224–6.

The Future of Homoeopathy. *Homoeopathy*, **21**, 157–60.

1972

Menopausal Depression. *British Homoeopathic Journal*, **61**, 3–11.

Homoeopathy and Psychosomatic Medicine. *General Practitioner*, 8 Jan., 9.

Asthma. *British Homoeopathic Journal*, **61**, 153–9.

Thuja and Chronic Virus Infection. *British Homoeopathic Journal*, **61**, 206–9.

Papers on Other Medical Subjects

1925

An Unusual Case of Supraclavicular Lymphadenitis. *Lancet*, **1**, 84.

1929

With A. L. Taylor. Portal Pyaemia following Diverticulitis. *Bristol Medico-Chirurgical Society Journal*, **46**, 131–40.

Indications for the Prescription of Dried Milks. *Medical Press and Circular*, **107**, 165.

1930

With Dr Paul Bodman. Perforation in Paratyphoid B. *Bristol Medico-Chirurgical Society Journal*, **47**, 316–21.

1934

Nervous Disorders in General Practice. *Bristol Medico-Chirurgical Society Journal*, **51**, 47–58.

1935

Nervous Disorders in General Practice. Abstract. *Medical Annual*, **53**, 284–6.

Publications

The Psychologic Background of Colitis. *American Journal of Medical Science*, **190**, 535 et seq. Abstract in *Zentralblatt f.d. Neurologie und Psychiatrie*, **55**, 223.

1937
The Role of the Central Nervous System in Disease. *Bristol Medico-Chirurgical Society Journal*, **54**, 41–63.

1941
With M. Dunsdon. Memorandum on Increase of Juvenile Delinquency in Wartime. *Lancet*, **2**, 572–4.

Reactions to Air-raid Warnings. *Lancet*, **1**, 177.

War Conditions and the Mental Health of the Child. *British Medical Journal*, **2**, 486–8.

1943
Clinic Statistics. *Times Educational Supplement*, 30 March, 33.

The Work of a Child Guidance Clinic. *National Froebel Foundation Bulletin*, March, 1–2.

Psychology in the Hospital Ward. *Nursing Times*, **39**, 540–5.

1945
With E. Stephens and L. K. Sambrook. Phantasies in Evacuated Children. *Journal of Mental Science*, **90**, 499–502.

Selection of Medical Students. *Bristol Medico-Chirurigical Society Journal*, Autumn, **62**.

Aggressive Play. *New Era Monograph, No. 3*, Nov. 1945.

Report: Bristol Child Guidance Clinic. *Annual Report of the School Medical Officer*, Bristol Education Committee, 9.

1946
Social Maturity Test. *Journal of Mental Science*, **91**, 532–41.

Psychiatric Cases Referred by Aftercare Officers in Region 7. *British Medical Journal*, 59–60.

The Integration of the Psychological Services under the New Education Act 1944. *Report of the Proceedings of a Conference on Mental Health*, 94–6.

The Treatment of Children in Hostels. *Report of Child Guidance Interclinic Conference, 1946*, 24–42.

1947
Spinal Pumping. *British Medical Journal*, **2**, 273–4.

1948
Enuresis. *British Medical Association and Magistrates Association*, May.

1949
Erziehungsprobleme in Italien, Oesterreich und England. *Basler Nachrichten*, 16 Sept.

Semaines Internationales d'Etudes pour l'Enfance Victimes de la Guerre. *Mental Health*, **9**, 43–4.

Friendships in Children's Homes. *Child Care Quarterly Review*, 117–19.

Publications

1950
Constitutional Factors in Institution Children. *Journal of Mental Science*, **96**, 245–53.
The Social Adaptation of Institution Children. *Lancet*, **1**, 173–6.
The Origins of Genius. *Lancet*, 549.
Constitutional Factors in Institution Children. *Digest of Neurology and Psychiatry*, **18**, 291.

1951
Some Administrative Problems of the Health Services. *Report of the Discussions of the March Conference*, 45–6.
Evidence. *Report of a Committee to Review Punishments in Prisons, Borstal Institutions, Approved Schools and Remand Homes*, Parts III and IV. H.M.S.O. Cmd 8429.

1952
Hostels for Maladjusted Children. *Report of the Chief Medical Officer of the Ministry of Education for the Years 1948 and 1949*, 68.

1953
Child Guidance. *Annual Report of the Principal School Medical Officer*. Somerset County Council, 16–18.
A Sociological Approach to Maladjustment. *Report on 10th Child Guidance Inter-Clinic Conference*. London, 44.

1958
Personal Factors in Problem Families. *Case Conference*, Sept., **5**.

1959
Obituary: Dr Sessions-Hodge. *British Medical Journal*, **2**, 157.
Guidance or Treatment. *British Medical Journal*, Dec., 23.

1961
Starting to Read. *Books*, 31.
School Phobia. *Annual Report of the Principal School Medical Officer*, Somerset County Council, 1960, 7.
Psychiatric Assessment of Juvenile Offenders. *Approved Schools Gazette*, **56**, 89–95.
Child Care and Child Guidance. *Case Conference*, **8**, 266–9.

1962
Parental Attitudes. *Annual Report of the Principal School Medical Officer*, Somerset County Council, 1961, 12–13.

1963
Classification of Juvenile Delinquents. *Bristol Medico-Chirurgical Society Journal*, **80**, 127–30.
Increase in Behaviour Disorders. *Annual Report of the Principal School Medical Officer*, Somerset County Council, 1962, 13.

1964
Too Permissive? *Annual Report of the Principal School Medical Officer*, Somerset County Council, 1963, 7–8.
Psychotherapy in Approved Schools. *Journal of Offender Therapy*, **9**, 37–40.
The Natural History of Detention. *Case Conference*, **12**, 220–2.

Index of Remedies

Abrotanum 103
Aconite 12, 23, 31, 40, 62, 103
Actaea Racemosa 61, 65, 73
Aesculus 73, 75, 76, 77
Aethusa 101, 103
Agaricus 52
Allium Cepa 111
Aloes 77, 111
Alumina 53, 62
Ambra Grisea 94
Antimony 84
Apis 47, 84, 85, 110
Argentum Nitricum 28, 48, 49, 58, 101
Arnica 30, 44, 52, 74, 76
Arsenicum Album 28, 32, 45, 47, 51, 58, 72, 80, 81, 84, 85, 90, 103, 110
Arsenicum Metallicum 23
Arum 73
Aurum 30, 50, 58

Baptisia 30, 52, 73
Barium 47
Baryta Carbonica 47, 55, 57
Belladonna 22, 31, 40, 51, 57, 93, 100
Bellis Perennis 94
Benzoic Acid 93, 110
Bryonia 23, 24, 27, 30, 47, 61, 63, 64, 65, 66, 95
Bufo 43

Calcarea Arsenica 51
Calcarea Carbonica 46, 57, 61, 62, 64, 65, 66, 69, 70, 107
Calendula 74
Camphor 22, 23, 24, 51, 68
Cannibis Indica 30

Capsicum 27, 28, 101, 102
Carbo Vegetabilis 48, 51
Carboneum Sulphuratum 47, 48
Caulophyllum 73
Causticum 31, 46, 50, 66, 98, 107
Chamomilla 27, 28, 39, 58, 68, 72, 81, 102, 103, 104
China 58, 60, 91
Cicuta 47, 58
Cimicifuga (see Actaea Racemosa)
Cina 67, 68, 69, 71, 104
Cinchona 75
Cobalt 55
Cocculus 50, 56, 88
Coffea 23, 91, 98
Collinsonia 73, 76, 78
Colocynth 61, 65
Conium 46
Cuprum Metallicum 24

Digitalis 27
Drosera 69
Dulcamara 27, 65, 66, 81

Eupatorium 73, 111

Ferrum Metallicum 72
Fluoric Acid 111

Gelsemium 24, 73
Glonoine 110
Graphites 69, 70, 107

Hamamelis 73, 74, 75, 77
Hepar Sulphuris 28, 41, 42, 92, 100
Hydrastis 73
Hyoscyamus 27, 31, 40, 51, 52
Hypericum 27

118

Ignatia 50, 55, 58, 72, 99, 100
Iodum 81
Ipecacuanha 80

Kali Bichromicum 65, 66
Kali Carbonicum 30, 79, 81, 82, 107
Kali Iodatum 65, 66
Kalmia 111

Lachesis 30, 33, 50, 51, 52, 60, 61, 89
Lathyrus 110
Laurocerasus 30
Ledum 65, 66
Lycopodium 31, 44, 46, 49, 55, 61, 65, 97, 98, 107

Mercurius 31, 48, 65, 66
Morbillinum 24, 82
Mezereum 66

Natrum Carbonicum 110
Natrum Muriaticum 49, 50, 55, 59, 61, 65, 107
Natrum Sulphuricum 30, 44, 81, 111
Nux Moschata 47, 52
Nux Vomica 12, 22, 23, 49, 58, 66, 72, 90, 99

Opium 52
Oxalic Acid 111

Paeonia 72, 74
Petroleum 52, 70, 85
Phosphoric Acid 50, 110
Phosphorus 27, 39, 46, 52, 53, 57, 78, 82, 89, 107

Phytolacca 66, 73
Platina 32, 49, 59
Plumbum Metallicum 52, 53, 55
Podophyllum 70, 71, 73, 111
Psorinum 49, 61, 81, 82, 85, 86, 93
Pulsatilla 12, 66, 72, 78, 80, 81, 84, 92, 96, 98, 100

Radium 63
Rhododendron 63
Rhus Toxicodendron 61, 62, 63, 64, 65, 66
Rumex 73
Ruta 61, 66

Sambucus 81, 82
Sanguinaria 73, 111
Secale 51, 52
Selenium 30
Sepia 30, 58, 61, 65, 90, 91, 107
Silica 32, 44, 46, 52, 61, 65, 81, 90, 97, 107, 110
Spongia 23, 39, 47, 81, 82
Staphysagria 50
Stramonium 31, 40, 51, 52, 60, 100
Sulphur 39, 40, 41, 42, 46, 48, 55, 56, 57, 58, 60, 61, 64, 65, 72, 90, 92, 94, 95

Tarentula 48
Thuja 98, 99

Verbascum 74
Veratrum Album 24, 51
Viscum 27

Classical Homoeopathy, Dr Margery Blackie, 1986. The complete teaching legacy of one of the most important homoeopaths of our time. 0906584140

Everyday Homoeopathy, Dr David Gemmell, 1987. A practical handbook for using homoeopathy in the context of one's own personal and family health care, using readily available remedies. 0906584183

Homoeopathic Prescribing, Dr Noel Pratt, revised 1985. A compact reference book covering 161 common complaints and disorders, with guidance on the choice of the appropriate remedy. 0906584035

Homoeopathy as Art and Science, Dr Elizabeth Wright Hubbard, 1990. The selected writings of one of the foremost modern homoeopaths.

0906584264

Homoeopathy in Practice, Dr Douglas Borland, reprinted 1988 with Symptom Index. Detailed guidance on the observation of symptoms and the choice of remedies. 090658406X

Insights into Homoeopathy, Dr Frank Bodman, 1990. Homoeopathic approaches to common problems in general medicine and psychiatry.

0906584280

Introduction to Homoeopathic Medicine (2nd Edition), Dr Hamish Boyd, 1989. A formal introductory text, written in categories that are familiar to the medical practitioner. 0906584213

Materia Medica of New Homoeopathic Remedies, Dr. O. A. Julian, paperback edition 1984. Full clinical coverage of 106 new homoeopathic remedies, for use in conjunction with the classical materia medicas. 0906584116

Studies of Homoeopathic Remedies, Dr Douglas Gibson, 1987. Detailed clinical studies of 100 major remedies. Well-known for the uniquely wide range of insights brought to bear on each remedy. 0906584175

Tutorials on Homoeopathy, Dr Donald Foubister, 1989. Detailed studies on a wide range of conditions and remedies. 0906584256

Medical and Nursing Books From Beaconsfield Publishers

Cardiovascular Problems in Practice, Dr Roger Blackwood, 1986. A practical guide to the management of the cardiological emergencies and problems that form part of the daily work of the non-specialist doctor.   0906584167

Disorders of Cardiac Rate, Rhythm and Conduction, Dr Hamish Watson, 1984. Detailed guidance on the use of the ECG in the diagnosis and management of the cardiac patient. Written for the general practitioner, hospital doctor and cardiac nurse.   0906584108

Handbook for Care, Muriel Flack, SRN and Margaret Johnston, RGN, 1986. A practical textbook for care assistants/nursing auxiliaries working in the community, in hospital or in the residential care sector.   0906584132

Herbal Medicine, Dr. R. F. Weiss, 1988. The leading textbook of medical herbalism. A systematic study of plant drugs within a framework of clinical diagnoses, with a wealth of suggested prescriptions.   0906584191

Hysterectomy and Vaginal Repair, Sally Haslett, SRN and Molly Jennings, MCSP, 1988. For the patient – explains these operations and how to prepare for them. Advice on what to do afterwards for a trouble-free return to normal life.   090658423X

Lymphoedema: Advice on Treatment, Dr Claud Regnard, Caroline Badger, SRN and Dr Peter Mortimer, 1988. For the patient – explains what lymphoedema is and provides a daily management plan that can be followed at home.   0906584248

Nursing for Continence, Christine Norton, SRN, 1986. The definitive text on the nursing care of the incontinent patient.   0906584159

Oral Morphine in Advanced Cancer (2nd Edition), Dr Roger Twycross and Dr Sylvia Lack, 1989. Explains in detail how to use oral morphine most effectively in the management of cancer pain.   0906584272

Oral Morphine: Information for Patients, Families and Friends, Dr Robert Twycross and Dr Sylvia Lack, 1988. Offers answers to questions frequently asked by cancer patients when advised to start morphine therapy.
          0906584221

Surgery and Your Heart, Mr Donald Ross and Barbara Hyams, 1982. Colour-illustrated booklet for patients facing, or who have recently had, heart surgery.
          0906584078

What Shall I Do? Questions and Answers in Cardiology, Dr Roger Blackwood and Dr Bev Daily, 1988. Questions from a GP and answers from a cardiologist on the cardiological queries that can be expected to arise in general practice.
          0906584205